Ronald J. Riegel D.V.M.

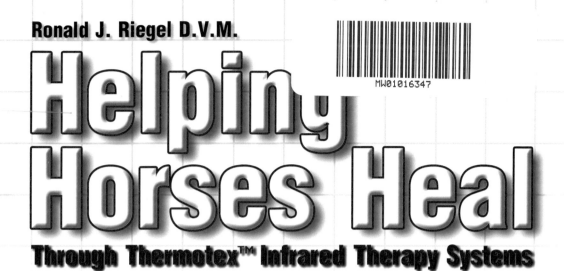

Helping Horses Heal
Through Thermotex™ Infrared Therapy Systems

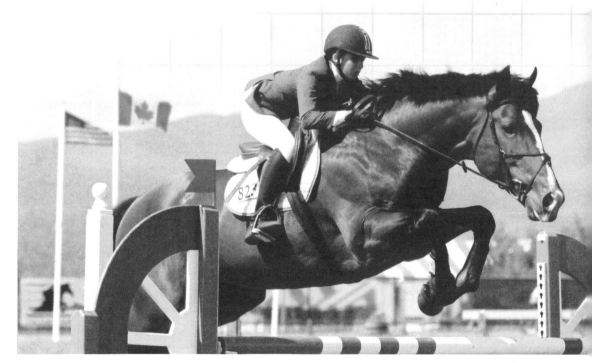

ISBN 0-9741845-1-9   Copyright © 2004 by Ronald J. Riegel D.V.M.

Disclaimer

The information and guidelines contained within this text have been collected through numerous years of use. To the best of our knowledge they are safe and effective in their applications to the equine species.

Veterinary consultation is essential for the equine athlete. Any injury or condition should be evaluated by the attending veterinarian before any type of physical therapy protocol is initiated. Each horse is an individual and results will vary depending on that animal's own unique physical characteristics.

Illustrated Animal Books Ltd.
18070 Raymond Rd.
Marysville, Ohio 43040

Better by Design
graphic design and production
www.bbdcreative.com

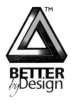

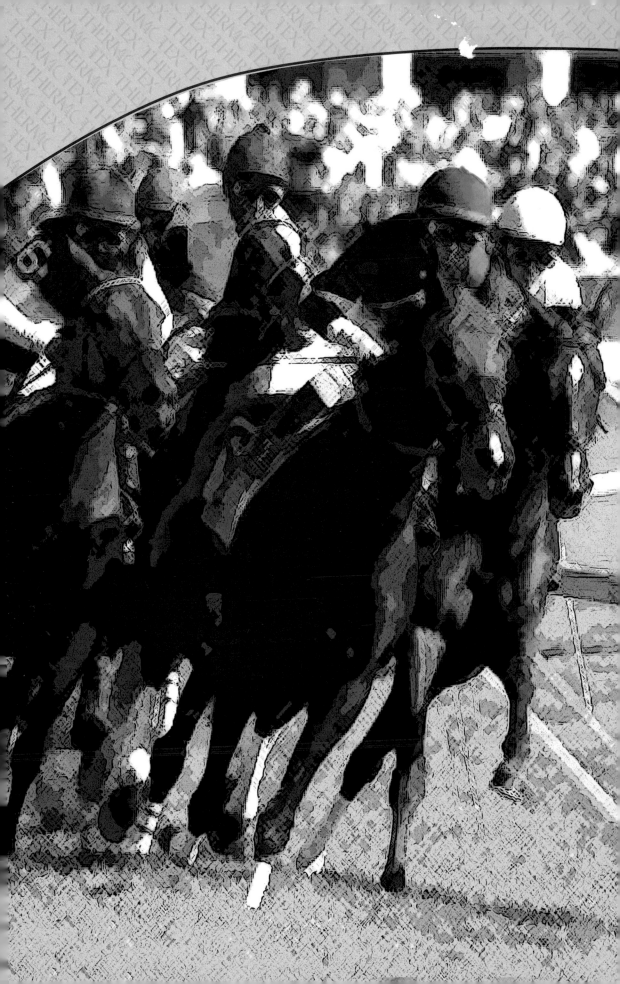

Table of Contents

Introduction

Why are the Thermotex™ Infrared Therapy
System Products so Unique? 01

Product Overview 02

How to Utilize this Text 02

Chapter One

The Therapeutic Benefits of Infrared Heat Therapy 05

What are the Effects of Infrared Therapeutic Heat Upon the
Physiologic Processes? 05

The Psychological Effect 06

Scientific Proof of the Thermotex™ Therapy System 06

Efficacy Study of the Thermotex™ Therapy System Infrared Heating Blanket
Upon the Standardbred Racehorse 07

Thermotex™ Therapy System Infrared Heating Pad
Versus a Conventional Heating Pad and a Hot Towel 18

Chapter Two

Basic Therapeutic Treatment Protocols Using the Thermotex™ Infrared Therapy Systems 23

Equipment and Patient Basics 24

Using the Thermotex™ Infrared Therapy System Blanket 25

General Use of the Hock and Legging Therapy Appliances 26

General Guidelines for the use of the Thermotex™ Infrared
Therapy System Neck Appliance 27

Guidelines for Using the Thermotex™ Infrared Therapy System
Hood Appliance 28

Table of Contents

Chapter Three

Therapy Protocols Using the Thermotex™ ITS Twelve Element Blanket 31

Pre-Event Warm-Up 31

Treatment of Clinical Disorders Utilizing the Thermotex™ ITS Blanket 35

Using the Thermotex™ ITS Blanket for the treatment of Secondary Compensatory Lameness 42

Utilization of the Thermotex™ ITS Blanket During the Training Regime for Prevention of Muscle Soreness 42

Using the Thermotex™ ITS Blanket as Part of a Total Therapy Program 44

Other Uses of the Thermotex™ ITS Blanket 46

Chapter Four

Basic Therapeutic Treatment Protocols Using the Thermotex™ ITS Extended Leggings 49

Equipment and Patient Basics when Using the Thermotex™ ITS Leggings 50

Using the Thermotex™ ITS Leggings as a Pre-Event Warm-Up 51

Using the Thermotex™ ITS Leggings as Treatment for Common Lameness ...51

Chapter Five

Basic Therapeutic Treatment Protocols Using the Thermotex™ ITS Neck Appliance 63

Equipment and Patient Basics when Using the Thermotex™ ITS Neck Appliance 64

Using the Thermotex™ ITS Neck Appliance as a Pre-Event Warm-Up 65

Using the Thermotex™ ITS Neck Appliance in a Daily Maintenance Program ..66

Using the Thermotex™ ITS Neck Appliance to Treat Various Disorders 66

Other Uses of the Thermotex™ ITS Neck Appliance 67

Chapter Six

Basic Therapeutic Treatment Protocols Using the Thermotex™ ITS Hood Appliance 69

Using the Thermotex™ ITS Hood Appliance for the Treatment of
Respiratory Disorders 70

Chapter Seven

Basic Therapeutic Treatment Protocols for TMJ Using the Thermotex™ ITS Hood 75

Temporomandibular Joint Function in the Horse 75

Temporomandibular Joint Anatomy and Function 78

Equine Dentistry 79

Therapeutic Effects 80

Basic Treatment Protocols 80

Chapter Eight

Basic Therapeutic Treatment Protocols Using the Thermotex™ ITS Appliances for each Discipline . .83

General Guidelines 84

General Guidelines for Using the Various Thermotex™ ITS Appliances for
Each Specific Discipline 85

Appendix A 101

Glossary 103

References 109

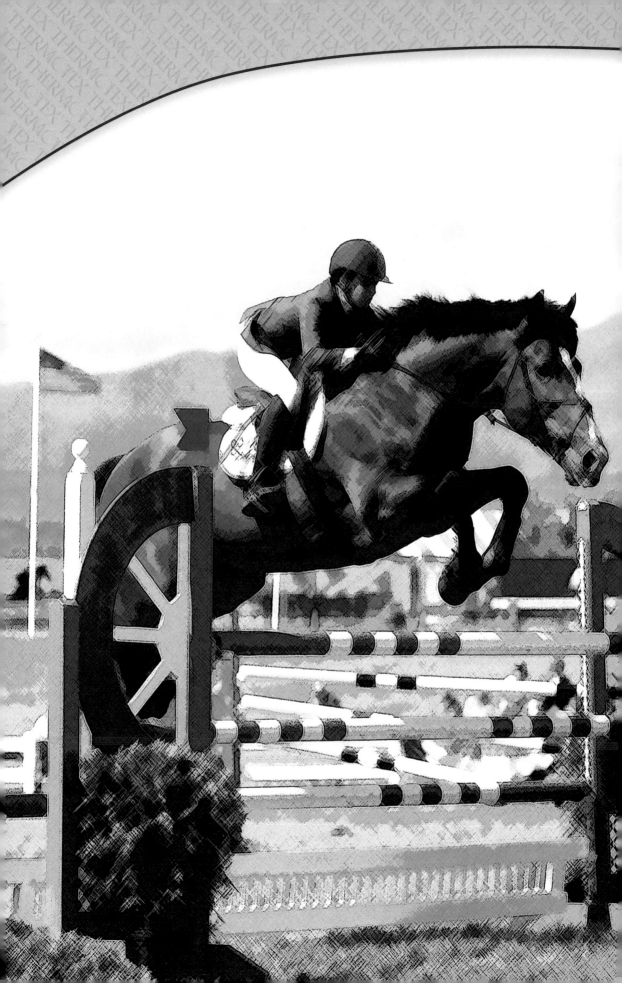

Introduction

The Goal of all Physical Therapy Modalities

The goal of all physical therapy modalities is to prevent injuries, increase athleticism or to return injured tissues to their pre-injury form and function. To accomplish this goal it is necessary to increase the circulation within the tissues. The application of heat has proven to be a fundamental method of achieving this goal.

Why are the Thermotex™ Therapy System Products so unique?

The Thermotex™ Therapy System provides a deep penetrating comfortable therapeutic heat that is significantly different from any other heating appliance on the market today. Each Thermotex™ Therapy System heating pad is constructed using the finest materials and utilizes deep penetrating infrared rays as the source of heat. This concept provides the Thermotex™ Therapy System with several distinct advantages over any other heating pad on the market.

- The Thermotex™ Therapy System delivers a more effective and relatively deep penetrating heat versus the conventional heating pads that rely on conductive heat production from wire coil resistance.

- Patients are comfortable during therapy since there is no overheating of the skin during treatment.

- Since there is no dehydration factor during treatment and there is a comforting application of heat, the Thermotex™ Therapy System can be applied for long periods of time, which optimizes the treatment.

- There are no adverse side effects during treatment such as burning or skin irritation.

- This deep therapeutic heat provided by the Thermotex™ Therapy System is relaxing to the patient and provides a comforting powerful psychological effect to the animal. Just watching the animals during and after treatment assures us that it must feel good to the animal.

About the cover
Momentous, an American Warmblood stallion, competes successfully with his 12 year old junior/amateur rider Ali Wolff.

" We have had great success with all of our Thermotex products. They are particularly helpful on our 17.2 hand stallion, Momentous. Our favorite product is the Thermotex blanket. We use the blanket at shows to expedite our warmup routine and for therapy when we return home. "
—Denise Phillips
Old Oak Farm
www.oldoakfarm.com

Product Overview:

Both conventional heating pads and the Thermotex™ Therapy System heating pads operate on 110 – 120V AC current. However, this is where the similarity ends. The Thermotex™ Therapy System heating pad radiates heat not from a live wire coil but from a unique and patented infrared element. Infrared heat waves are produced via a long wave of low frequency in the 9-12 micron range.

The physical structure of the Thermotex™ Therapy System heating pads and the production of infrared heat waves allow for a deep penetrating heat without the uncomfortably hot feeling of a conventional heating pad. There is very little conduction of heat from the Thermotex™ Therapy System heating pad but there is substantial radiated heat. This unique heating system allows comfortable treatment for extended periods of time to the patient.

Conventional heating pads that rely on wire resistance to produce conductive heat create very little radiated heat. The wavelengths of the conducted heat produced in this manner are very short and do not penetrate to any appreciable depth. Therefore, the possibility exists to dehydrate the skin tissues and even burn or irritate the skin.

Within a few applications, the patient, your horse, will experience a difference with the deep penetrating Thermotex™ Therapy System heating pads regardless of their athletic endeavor.

How to Utilize this Text:

Each horse is an individual and should be evaluated and treated in their own unique manner. This text will serve as a guideline for the numerous fundamental uses of the Thermotex™ Therapy System products. It is important to obtain an accurate diagnosis before initiating any treatment protocol regardless of the treatment modality.

Guidelines will be presented in the general use of the Thermotex™ Therapy System products. Various disorders will be discussed in brief terms with broad applications of the Thermotex™ Therapy System products.

The Thermotex™ Therapy System product line:

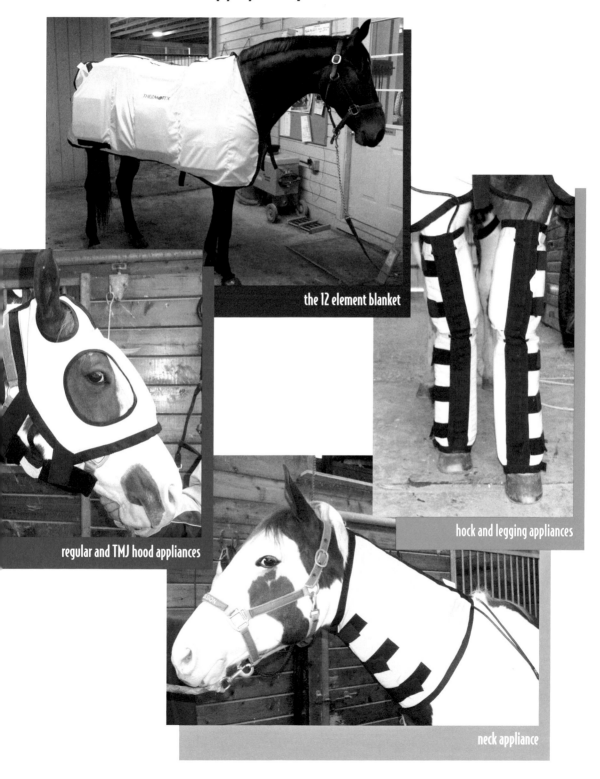

the 12 element blanket

regular and TMJ hood appliances

hock and legging appliances

neck appliance

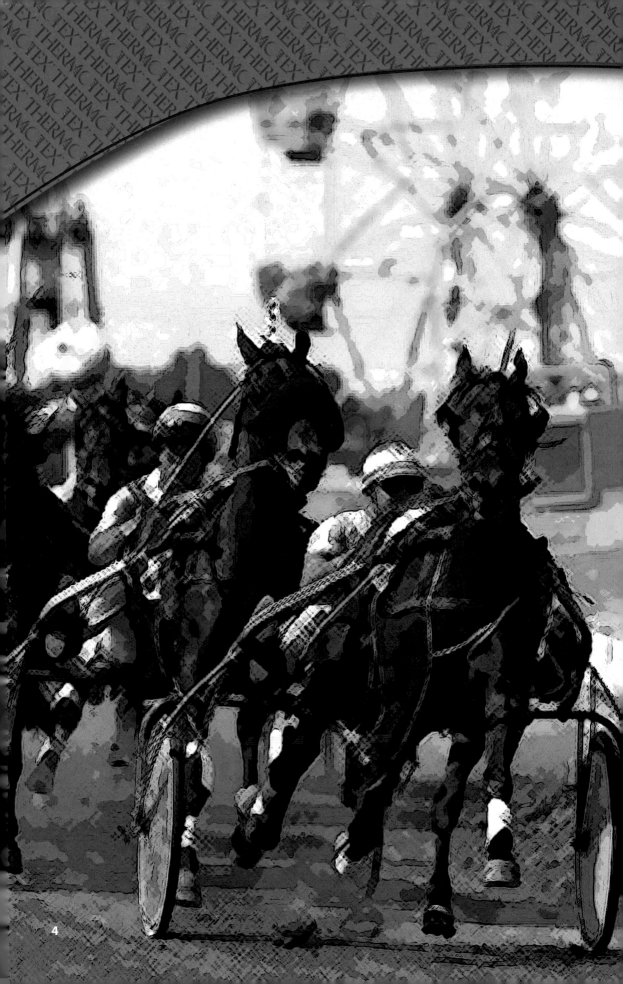

The Therapeutic Benefits of Infrared Heat Therapy

What are the effects of infrared therapeutic heat upon the physiological processes?

Infrared therapeutic heat provides a deep penetrating form of thermal energy. This increase in thermal energy within the tissues results in an increase in the metabolic processes within the cells. Therefore, there is an increase in the blood flow to the area, a decrease in pain, a decrease in stiffness and an increase in tissue extensibility.

The increase in metabolic activity within the cells results in an increased demand for oxygen and a resultant *vasodilatation* or increased blood flow to the area. This increase in blood flow is usually six times that of the blood flow to the same anatomical area during resting conditions. This increase in circulation not only brings more oxygen to the area but also supplies the area with more nutrients and provides a means to remove the cellular waste products created during repair.

Did you know?

Infrared heat has an analgesic effect on tissue and provides a sedative effect upon the sensory nerve endings.

Application of infrared heat also has an *analgesic* effect upon the tissues. Infrared heat provides a sedative effect upon the sensory nerve endings. This ultimately leads to a relaxation within the tissues especially the muscle tissues. As a result of the increase in circulation, the waste products of injury such as *prostaglandins*, *bradykinin* and *histamine* are removed at an increased rate and are not allowed to stay in the area creating nerve fiber sensitization and pain. The application of heat results in an overstimulation of the nervous tissue in that there is an increased ability for the nerve to receive and transmit impulses. This overstimulation interferes with the nerve fibers' ability to perceive pain therefore resulting in a state of analgesia.

An increase in the blood flow and by increasing the temperature within, muscle tissue elasticity is enhanced. Muscles become relaxed and are not in a state of spasm. This permits them to elongate further and more efficiently when placed under exercise load. When heat is applied to tendons and ligaments, they become more elastic and flexible thusly providing some prevention to strains and sprains while exercising.

Infrared heat allows tendons and ligaments to be more flexible.

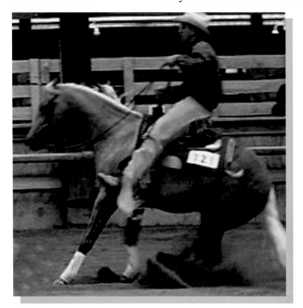

Providing deep penetrating infrared thermal energy to a joint has numerous benefits. There is an immediate increase within the elasticity and flexibility of the tendons and ligaments associated with that joint. This allows a greater range of motion and a relief of stiffness. There is a decrease within the *viscosity* of the *synovial* fluid within the joint allowing it to function in an enhanced state of lubrication. Analgesia to the joint is accomplished through the same mechanisms described above.

The Psychological Effect.

Using Thermotex™ Therapy System Products upon the equine athlete has many psychological benefits. Observation of the patient indicates that it feels good to the animal. After the first few minutes of the Thermotex™ Therapy System Infrared Therapy Blanket the animal can be seen lowering its head and relaxing. Often its eyes will begin to close and its stance will become increasingly relaxed.

When the Therapy Blanket is used as a pre-event warm-up, the benefits of this relaxed psychological state can be realized. The animal will be able to perform at the peak of its athletic ability having been relieved of its stress and returned to a more limber state.

The relief of pain also has a powerful psychological effect. If the equine athlete suffers from sore muscles and this is relieved through the use of the Thermotex™ Therapy System Products, they will function at a higher level within their discipline. "A pain free horse is a happy horse and a happy horse usually will perform to their fullest athletic potential."

Scientific Proof of the Thermotex™ Therapy System.

Several studies have been completed to substantiate the efficacy of the Thermotex™ Therapy System Products. How sad that more of the physical therapy devices on the market for both equine and human athletes have not had the same authentication.

EFFICACY STUDY OF THE THERMOTEX™ INFRARED HEATING BLANKET UPON THE STANDARDBRED RACEHORSE

RONALD J. RIEGEL D.V.M.

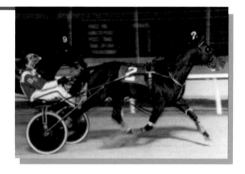

HYPOTHESIS:

Harness racing is one of the most demanding of all of the equine athletic endeavors. Months of foundation miles are accomplished before this athlete is even close to race condition and speed. After this long period of training, the animal must then drop in time, over the mile distance, to be competitive. This hard training regime is extremely taxing upon the equine athlete and all methods must be considered to alleviate the pain and inflammation within the musculature to ensure the success of this equine athlete.

> " The application of infrared heat to the equine athlete allows for an increase in exercise efficiency of at least 10%. "
>
> –Dr. Ronald Reigel,
> *The Illustrated Atlas of Equine Anatomy and Common Disorders of the Horse*

The Thermotex™ Infrared Therapy Blanket has been scientifically proven to be effective in providing deep heat to the musculature of the equine athlete. Infrared thermographs correlated with blood chemistry analysis will provide proof that this physical therapy modality is effective in relieving inflammation within the muscle tissues of these equine athletes.

INFRARED HEAT AS A PHYSICAL THERAPY MODALITY:

The application of infrared heat to the animal in itself possesses many benefits. Application to the muscle tissues provides vasodilatation of the blood vessels, an increased circulation of blood and lymph, an increased metabolic rate within the tissues, a reduction in swelling and consequentially, a reduction in inflammation within the musculature. These therapeutic benefits aid in both the restoration and healing within these muscle tissues, allowing for an increase in potential athletic ability and speeding the recovery of the entire athlete from an arduous training schedule.

GOALS:

These are the questions that will be answered by this research endeavor:

1. Will the infrared thermal gradients within the musculature of the lumbar and sacral spinal anatomical areas be reduced when treatment with the Thermotex™ Infrared Therapy Blanket is applied?

2. What are the clinical pathological changes within the blood chemistry levels as an animal receives treatment with the Thermotex™ Infrared Therapy Blanket?

3. Will there be a correlation between the thermographic findings and the blood serum chemistry findings?

INFRARED THERMOGRAPHY:

An infrared thermograph is a pictorial representation of the surface temperature of the anatomical area it is measuring. The circulatory system, inflammation, environmental changes, the metabolic rate of the animal and other unique individual thermographic characteristics influence its measurements.

A thermographic workstation.

The use of infrared thermography as a measurement of the efficacy of different therapeutic modalities is easily accomplished. Changes within thermal gradients can depict a decrease or increase in circulation, a decrease or increase in inflammation and even nerve irritation some-where along the neuron pathway. Therapeutic results can be visualized by a series of infrared thermographs taken over a period of time and then compared.

BLOOD CHEMISTRY ANALYSIS:

AST is an abbreviation for Aspartate aminotransferase, which is the synonym for the antiquated term SGOT (serum glutamic oxaloacetic transaminase). This enzyme occurs in almost all cells within the body but it is used to primarily diagnose liver and muscle disease. The liver and muscle cells have the highest activity of this enzyme. In itself it is not specific for a liver disorder but is more diagnostic for the muscle tissues.

Aspartate aminotransferase is present in the mitochondria and the cytoplasmic fluid within the cells. The serum levels of this enzyme are increased following hard exercise or skeletal muscle injury. Circulating concentrations of this enzyme will peak approximately 24 hours after an inciting incident and return to normal within 7 – 10 days.

CPK (CK) is an abbreviation for Creatine phosphokinase (or Creatine kinase). This is the most organ-specific of all of the clinical enzymes. Most serum CPK activity is from a muscu-lar origin. The plasma half-life of this enzyme is short and will peak as early as six hours. This enzyme will take 2 - 3 days to return to normal levels.

PROCEDURE AND METHODOLOGY:

Two groups of ten, three and four-year-old standardbred racehorses, that are in full training will be used as the test subjects. These twenty animals will have to meet the fol-lowing criteria:

These animals will be healthy upon physical examination.

The animals will be serviceably sound and not had any or be given any systemic or intraarticular medications. This includes all steroidal and nonsteroidal anti-inflammatory medications such as phenylbutazone, flunixin meglumine and corticosteroids.

Training schedules and racing times are all similar and near-ly in the same class of races.

Did you know?

Infrared thermography was developed by the defense department in the 1950s. Medical applications in the human field originated in the 1970s.

All other physical therapy modalities and topical applications of counterirritants discontinued at least seven days before the initiation of this project.

The study will last six weeks, have a two-week break to all equine subjects and then resume with the control group becoming the treatment group and the treatment group becoming the control group for another six weeks.

All twenty animals will be thermographed initially, and then at weekly intervals during the duration of the study. Blood samples will be taken initially from all of the animals and then repeated weekly until the conclusion of the study. These blood samples will be evaluated for a complete blood count and total serum chemistry analysis.

The complete blood count will have the following parameters tested:

- RBC count
- WBC count
- Packed cell volume
- The types of WBC's
- Normal hematology.

The serum chemistry analysis included:

- Albumin levels: 35 – 50% of the serum protein.
- Alkaline Phosphatase levels: hepatic function.
- BUN: renal function
- Calcium: calcium metabolism
- Creatinine: renal function
- Glucose: measured to monitor other diseases
- Magnesium: magnesium metabolism
- Phosphorus: phosphorus metabolism
- AST (SGOT)
- Serum protein: nutritive function
- Total bilirubin: hepatic function
- Sodium: electrolyte balance
- Potassium: electrolyte balance
- Chloride: electrolyte balance
- GGT: renal function

- CPK (CK)
- A/G ratio: albumin/globulin ratio; total protein values
- Globulin: calculated by subtracting the albumin concentration from the total protein concentration.
- Lipemic index: hepatic function
- Hemolytic index: a value that may affect other tests.
- Icteric index: hepatic function.

The animals were randomly placed into two groups: a treatment group and a control group.

Those animals within the control group did not receive any treatments with the Thermotex™ Infrared Therapy Blanket during that portion of the study. The animals within the treatment group received treatments for thirty minutes each day just before exercise. The temperature control was placed on the high setting for ten minutes and then on the low setting for the remaining twenty-minute duration of the treatment.

Thermographs and blood samples were taken before exercise every seven days for fourteen weeks.

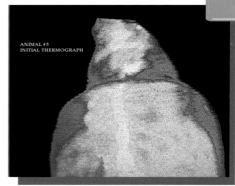

Initial thermograph—animal #5.

RESULTS AND DISCUSSION:

Thermographic Results:

The initial infrared thermograph (See initial thermograph – animal #5) revealed an increased thermal gradient over the thoracic, lumbar and lumbosacral spine. This thermograph was taken at a setting of 0.5 degrees centigrade per isothermic level. White is the highest reading and purple is the coldest or lowest level with a five-degree difference between them. These areas depicted by the color white were fairly symmetrical except within the lumbosacral area. In this anatomical area, there is an increased thermal gradient predominantly on the left side. These areas of white, gold and yellow reveal an increased thermal gradient within the tissues that is indicative of an inflammatory response within.

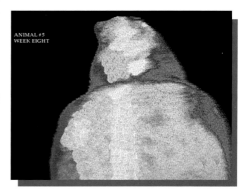

Infrared Thermograph Week 8—animal #5.

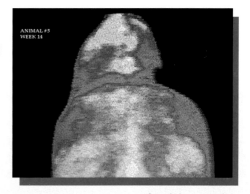

Infrared Thermograph Week 14—animal #5.

This particular animal (#5) was chosen as an example of the entire study since the response within this animal was close to the average of animals within the entire study. This animal also palpated digitally with a slight tenderness throughout the areas that are depicted by the color white.

After eight weeks of training without any treatment, the infrared thermograph of animal number five revealed the following comparisons to the initial thermograph. (See infrared thermograph – animal #5 – week 8) There is an increase within all of the thermal gradients as compared to the initial findings. The increased thermal gradients throughout the thoracic spine now continue into the right shoulder region. Those increased thermal gradients within the lumbar and lumbosacral areas have increased in intensity and are now more predominant on the left side continuing into the gluteal areas. These increases are due to a rigorous training schedule and are normal for an animal that is receiving no therapeutic help for this inflammation.

All ten of the animals that were in the control group depicted these types of thermographs for the first eight weeks of the study. They were all becoming increasingly sore and their thermographs all revealed increases along the lumbar and sacral spine.

Immediately after treatment with the Thermotex™ Infrared Therapy Blanket, there was a huge increase within the thermal gradients within the tissues. This increase lasted an average of four to five hours after the treatment was concluded. These thermographs were done before the initiation of the study just to establish a baseline of data. During the study, the animals were always exercised after their treatment, which also increased the thermal gradients found within the individual making the duration of the effect impossible to measure.

The infrared thermograph taken of animal #5 at the conclusion of the study revealed large decreases within the thermal gradients along all of the anatomical areas examined. (See infrared thermograph – week 14) Within the lumbosacral spine area there is a remarkable 95% reduction within the thermal gradients. Clinically this also corresponds to insensitivity upon digital palpation. The thoracic

> " I love my Thermotex Blankets. I have several training stables at different tracks and all of my trainers use the infrared blankets to achieve the best results.
>
> Dick Clark is one of my leading trainers at Prairie Meadows each year. He uses three blankets to keep his horses in great racing shape. "
>
> – Maggie Moss

and thoracolumbar spinal areas also experienced a reduction within the thermal gradients to an extent of 68% reduction. This area was also no longer sensitive to digital palpation.

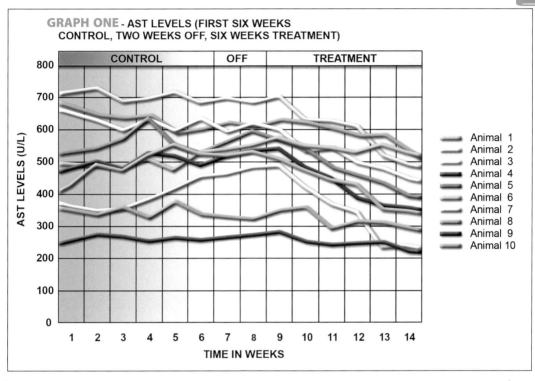

GRAPH ONE - AST LEVELS (FIRST SIX WEEKS CONTROL, TWO WEEKS OFF, SIX WEEKS TREATMENT)

Graph One

Serum Chemistry Results:

The AST levels for the ten animals that served in the control group were consistently high during the first eight weeks of the study and then gradually dropped to lower levels during the last six weeks of the study. *(See graph one)*

Initially, seven of the ten animals tested with higher than normal AST levels within the serum. By week eight, eight of the ten animals depicted AST levels higher than normal. After the initiation of treatment at week eight, these levels gradually fell, in all but those animals testing normally, to a level lower than that found at the eight week tests. By week fourteen, six of the ten animals were now testing within normal limits. The results seen within graph one summarize this data.

Those animals that initially received treatment for six weeks and then were left untreated revealed quite different results within their AST levels. *(See graph two)*

Five of these ten animals depicted higher than normal AST levels at the initiation of treatment. Nine of the ten animals experienced an immediate drop within the first week of treatment. By week six, seven of the ten animals were testing within normal AST ranges. After the cessation of treatments, seven of the ten animals within this group immediately experienced a rise within the AST levels during

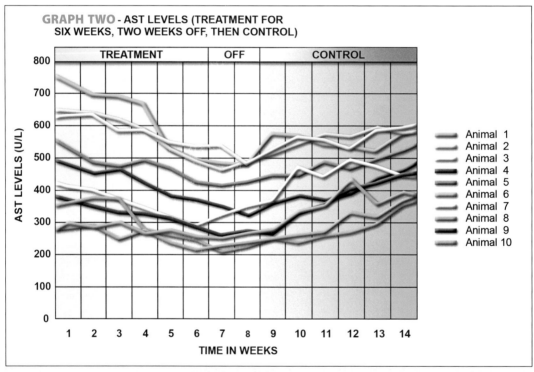

GRAPH TWO - AST LEVELS (TREATMENT FOR SIX WEEKS, TWO WEEKS OFF, THEN CONTROL)

Graph Two

week seven. At fourteen weeks, eight of the ten animals revealed higher AST levels than those measured initially. The data charted on graph two reveals this decline in AST levels through week six and then a gradual increase when the use of the Thermotex™ Infrared Therapy Blanket was stopped.

The CK levels followed the same pattern as the AST levels within the group of ten animals that was used as a control for eight weeks and then provided treatment. *(See graph three)*

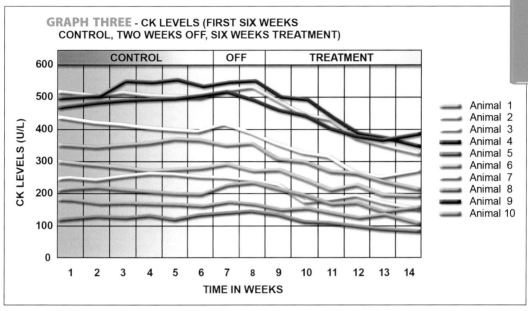

GRAPH THREE - CK LEVELS (FIRST SIX WEEKS
CONTROL, TWO WEEKS OFF, SIX WEEKS TREATMENT)

Graph Three

Initially, five of the ten animals tested within the normal limits for CK levels in the horse. By week eight, six of the animals tested with an increase in CK levels over those initial levels. Over the next six weeks, during treatment with the Thermotex™ Infrared Therapy Blanket, all ten of the animals experienced a decline in CK levels. Eight of the ten animals are now testing within normal limits. The other two animals could even be considered in the high normal range.

Graph three is a summary of all of the averages on a weekly basis. During the control part of the study, the group maintained an even level throughout the first 6-8 weeks. After the initiation of treatment, the CK levels gradually fell.

When the animals initially received treatment and then became the control group, the results mimicked those of the same AST group. *(See graph four)*

Initially, only four of the ten animals tested within normal limits for CK. After six weeks of treatment with the Thermotex™ Infrared Therapy Blanket, six of the ten animals were within normal limits. By the time fourteen weeks had passed, seven of the ten animals exhibited higher than normal levels with seven of the ten animals also showing increased levels from the initial testing. Graph four exhibits

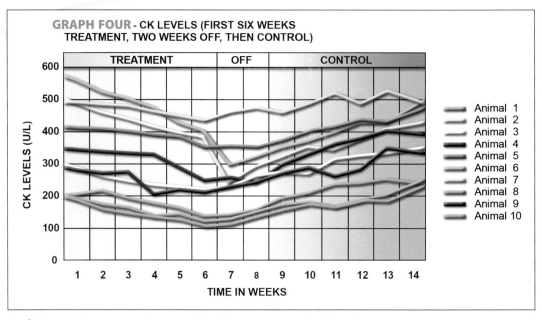

Graph Four

the gradual decline in CK levels and then the gradual increase after treatment protocols have ceased.

The summary of the blood chemistry analysis revealed that the AST and CK levels were lower during treatment with the Thermotex™ Infrared Therapy Blanket. *(See graph five)*

As depicted in the graphs, the AST and CK levels increased while the animals were in training and not receiving treatment with the Thermotex™ Infrared Therapy Blanket and decreased when receiving treatment.

For more graphs showing data averages see Appendix A.

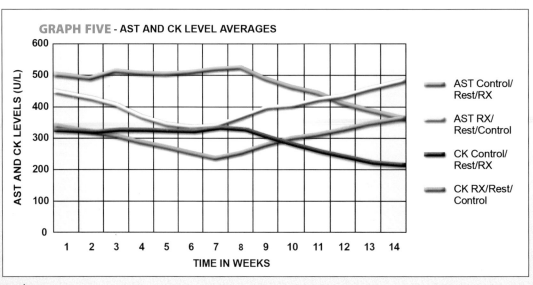

Graph Five

SUMMARY AND CONCLUSIONS:

The evidence provided by this study allows the following conclusions:

There are both thermographic and serum chemistry evidence that the infrared heat therapy provided by the Thermotex™ Infrared Therapy Blanket is efficacious.

The lowering of both the AST and CK levels indicates that treatment with the Thermotex™ Infrared Therapy Blanket alleviates the inflammatory response within the muscles of the standard-bred racehorses that are in training.

Thermographic evidence provides evidence of a decrease within the inflammatory response when the Thermotex™ Infrared Therapy Blanket is used on a daily basis.

This study concludes that the Thermotex™ Infrared Therapy Blanket is a drug free physical therapy modality that is efficacious before competition, as a therapy program in itself, as an adjunct to other physical therapy modalities such as massage, as a preventive program for athletic injuries and as a tool to help improve the quality of life for the equine athlete.

REFERENCES:

Bromiley, Mary. Physiotherapy in Veterinary Practice. Blackwell Scientific Publications Editorial Offices. 1991. Pg. 16-21.

Riegel, Ronald and Hakola, Susan. *Illustrated Atlas of Clinical Equine Anatomy and Common Disorders of the Horse.* Equistar Publications Ltd. 1996.

Stashak, S. Ted. *Adam's Lameness in Horses.* Fourth Edition. Lea and Febiger. 1987. Philadelphia. 1962.

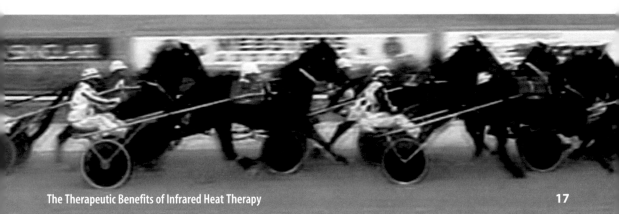

THERMOTEX™ THERAPY SYSTEM INFRARED HEATING PAD VERSUS A CONVENTIONAL HEATING PAD AND A HOT TOWEL

RONALD J. RIEGEL D.V.M.

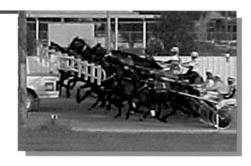

HYPOTHESIS:

Many consider the hindquarters and especially the gluteal muscles the "engine" of the horse. Intense, high level training places great physical demands upon these muscles. Standardbred racehorses not only have to have speed but also endurance and stamina. This breed of horse, because of the training regimes utilized, places an incredible amount of stress upon these muscle tissues.

Traditionally, placing a hot towel, then an electric heating pad and then a stable blanket, to hold all of this in place, is the standard treatment for muscle soreness in this area. This system, although cumbersome, does have some degree of success but how deep does the heat really go? Does the Thermotex™ Therapy System Heating pad provide an easier and deeper penetrating heat to this anatomical area?

> " I have been a Thermotex distributor for a number of years and have over 128 satisfied clients in six different states. Many of these trainers use up to four Thermotex blankets in their training programs. "
>
> –John Michaluk

GOALS:

These are the questions that will be answered by this endeavor:

How deep within the tissue will the heat from the traditional hot towel/electric heating pad penetrate?

How deep within the tissue will the Thermotex™ Therapy System Infrared heating pad penetrate?

Will there be any side effects such as skin soreness, pain or dehydration with the traditional treatment?

Will there be any side effects such as skin soreness, pain or dehydration using the Thermotex™ Therapy System Infrared heating pad?

PROCEDURE AND METHODOLOGY:

Two four-year-old standardbred racehorses were chosen at random. Both animals had to meet the following criteria:

Both animals were in good health and free of any visible signs of lameness.

No medication, systemic, intraarticular or topical, had been administered to the animals within the preceeding three weeks.

The level of training was similar for each animal.

Over the past two weeks, no other physical therapy modalities were administered to them.

Each of the equine subjects will serve as their own control. A thermocouple probe will be placed at varying depths within the musculature. On the right side of the gluteal area a Thermotex™ Therapy System heating pad will be used to treat the musculature whereas on the left side the traditional treatment of a warm moist towel covered by a heating pad will be used.

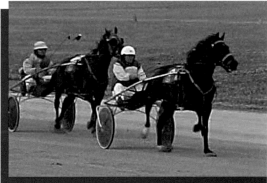

Two four-year-old standardbred racehorses were chosen at random.

Thermocouples will be placed at 1/2 centimeter intervals to a depth of six centimeters. The first will be placed just beneath the skin. The remainder will be placed centrally within the gluteus medius muscle at the stated depths.

Therapy will last twenty minutes with both the electric heating pad and the Thermotex™ Therapy System infrared heating pad set at their highest settings. Temperatures will be recorded at five minute intervals at each depth.

RESULTS AND DISCUSSION:

The literature states that the muscle tissue must rise at least five degrees to increase the metabolic rate of the muscle cells. There is a "therapeutic window," with the application of heat, where it is beneficial and not at a level that is causing pain.

The normal skin temperature of the horse is approximately 90° Fahrenheit. Therefore, the source of heat to the tissues must be greater than this level to increase the underlying tissue temperatures. Application of temperatures greater than 133° Fahrenheit, for a prolonged period of time, will cause skin sensitivity and eventually damage to the dermis. Gentle deep penetrating heat is ideal therapy for this muscle tissue.

Data was collected and revealed the following results:

The Thermotex™ Therapy System infrared heating pad achieved both a higher level of temperature within the tissues and a greater depth of penetration within the musculature.

The temperature of the musculature rose faster and stayed at a therapeutic level longer with the Thermotex™ Therapy System infrared heating pad than using the conventional heating pad and a hot towel.

Upon digital palpation there wasn't any soreness or pain elicited by either treatment.

If there was any dehydration by either treatment, it was minimal.

For data on depth of temperature penetration see Appendix B.

> " Master Joe has raced since his 2 year-old year. Since his 4 year-old year, he has had the benefits of the therapeutic infrared Thermotex™ blanket. After only 2 months of using the blanket, Master Joe ran his personal best, 153²/⁵ at Scioto Downs. "
> – Russel Angelbeck

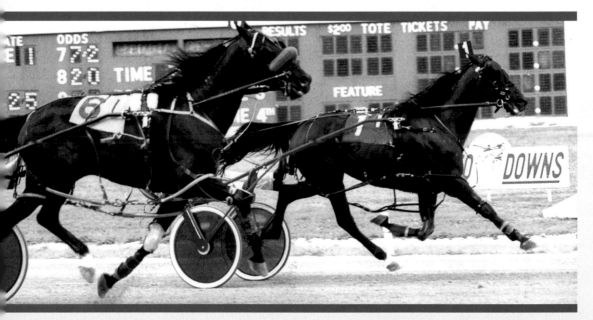

SUMMARY AND CONCLUSIONS:

The scientific evidence provided by this study allows the following conclusions:

The Thermotex™ Therapy System infrared heating pads provide a very therapeutic, deep penetrating form of heat to the musculature.

The temperature within the muscle tissue rises faster and is maintained at a therapeutic level longer when compared to the conventional therapy.

REFERENCES:

Bromiley, Mary. Physiotherapy in Veterinary Practice. Blackwell Scientific Publications Editorial Offices. 1991. Pg. 16-21.

Riegel, Ronald and Hakola, Susan. Illustrated Atlas of Clinical Equine Anatomy and Common Disorders of the Horse. Equistar Publications Ltd. 1996.

Sisson, S.B. Septimus and Grossman, D. James. The Anatomy of the Domestic Animals. W. B Saunders Company. Philadelphia.

Stashak, S. Ted. Adam's Lameness in Horses. Fourth Edition. Lea and Febiger. 1987. Philadelphia. 1962.

Master Joe is an 8 year-old Standardbred that has raced since his 2 year-old year. In 112 lifetime starts he has 17 wins, 8 second, and 18 thirds for a lifetime earnings of $63,317.00.

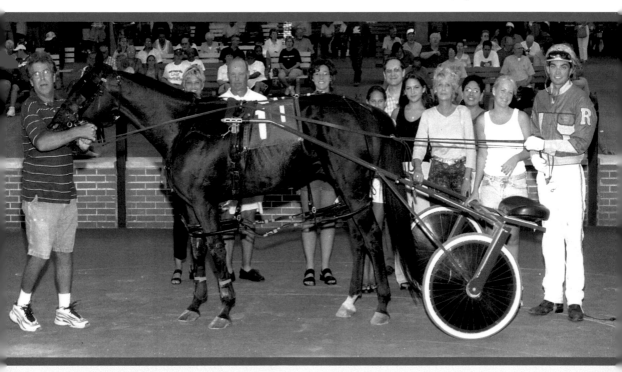

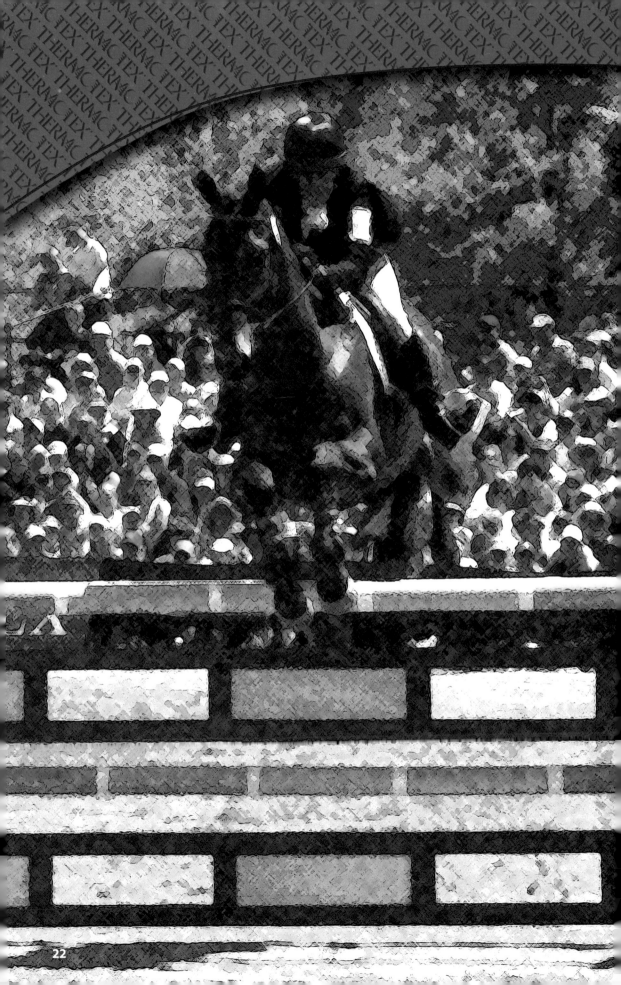

CHAPTER TWO

Basic Therapeutic Treatment Protocols Using the Thermotex™ Infrared Therapy Systems

Introduction:

The following physiological effects are the result of the application of infrared therapeutic heat:

- *Vasodilatation* and increased blood flow.
- *Analgesia*.
- Increased metabolic activity within the cells.
- Increased tissue extensibility.
- Decrease in joint stiffness.

Did you know?

The goal of any physical therapy modality is to increase the blood flow to a specific area and either restore or increase the function of the target tissues.

To achieve these desired physiological effects, the application of infrared therapeutic heat and the duration of treatment must be accurate.

Several basic measures must be undertaken for this **modality** to have the maximum effectiveness. If the Thermotex™ Infrared Therapy System is used as a treatment modality, an accurate diagnosis of the problem is needed before treatment is initiated. If the Thermotex™ Infrared Therapy System is used as a pre-event procedure, the type of discipline the equine athlete is involved in will dictate how the equipment should be utilized to maximize performance. If the Thermotex™ Infrared Therapy System is used to prevent injuries on a routine basis, this is yet another topic with its own unique characteristics.

Equipment and Patient Basics:

The patient should have its head tied up and ideally be in cross-ties. The animal should be clean and not have any dirt or other material, such as a poultice, on the area to be treated. Brushing the animal is always a good idea before placing the Thermotex™ Infrared Therapy System blanket upon the horse for therapy. If cross-ties are not available, it is a good idea to muzzle the animal before placing any of the products on the horse for *therapy*.

The entire Thermotex™ Infrared Therapy System is dependent upon electricity. Plug any of the appliances into a 110V/120V outlet before placing on the horse to pre-warm it. Application to the horse is then more comfortable for the animal and it prevents the initial chill from a cold blanket that could spasm sore muscles even further.

After application of any of the Thermotex™ Infrared Therapy System products, make sure all of the electric cords are out of reach of the patient. Remember, the cords must not only be away from the animal's mouth but also away from any contact with their metal shoes. Toe grabs and caulks will easily penetrate an electric cord, which may lead to electrocution for the patient.

Never use anything underneath the Thermotex™ Infrared Therapy System pads. Warm moist towels do not amplify the therapy achieved from the system. Liniments, sweats, counterirritants and any topical applications of any substance should be avoided. You may get an adverse reaction to these substances that will result in an irritation to the skin. The treatment area should be clean, dry and free of any substance.

The Thermotex™ Infrared Therapy blanket in use.

Using the Thermotex™ Infrared Therapy System Blanket:

The Thermotex Infrared Therapy System is the best heat producing therapy device on the market and it is important that you use it properly to achieve maximum results.

The following is an easy general step-by-step procedure that should be followed each time the blanket is used:

1. With the temperature setting on high, plug the blankct in and allow it to pre-warm for at least five minutes.

2. Unplug the blanket and place the blanket on the horse.

3. Fasten it securely with all of the Velcro straps to fit smartly on the patient.

4. Plug the blanket into a good extension cord making sure that the cords are all out of reach of the horse's head and all four feet.

5. Start the therapy session with the temperature setting on high for at least 10 to 15 minutes.

6. Check all of the pads and confirm that the pads are in the desired pockets.

7. After at least 20 minutes the infrared heating pads can be moved within the pockets to further treat that anatomical area.

8. Most therapy sessions should last a minimum of 30 minutes but when treating a clinical condition, therapy can last at least one hour or more.

9. After the therapy session, remove the blanket, wipe clean with a disinfecting cloth and allow to dry completely before storing.

10. Use a light to medium towel to dry any areas of perspiration and lightly massage any areas of soreness.

Long therapy sessions are not uncommon when using the Thermotex™ Infrared Therapy System blanket. The patented infrared pads will not overheat the tissues and will not cause the *dehydration* of any of the body fluids from the patient. In cases of severe *myositis*, the Thermotex™ Infrared Therapy System blanket has been used up to eight hours, in a 24-hour period, in a cold climate with only beneficial results to the patient.

General Use of the Hock and Legging Therapy Appliances:

Anatomically, the areas of the knee and hock and distally down the limb are composed of tendons and *ligaments* with very little muscle tissue present. Infrared heat therapy to these areas will allow more tendon and ligament extensibility and benefit all of the joints in this area. These joints will be relieved of stiffness and have a greater range of motion post treatment.

If a clinical problem exists, an accurate diagnosis should be attained before the initiation of treatment. An acute swollen flexor tendon is an example of a case that requires immediate diagnosis. If the injury is only a few hours old, infrared heat therapy would most likely be the wrong approach to take.

The following general step-by-step guidelines should be followed when using these therapy appliances:

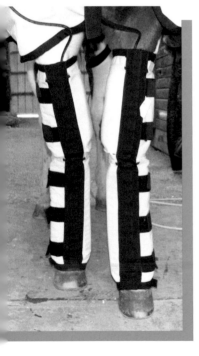

The Thermotex™ Infrared Therapy leggings in use.

1. Plug in the Thermotex™ Infrared Therapy System legging appliance to pre-warm for a few minutes.

2. Restrain the animal so neither its mouth or feet will come in contact with any of the electric cords. Cross-ties work well.

3. Make sure the leg is completely free of liniments, sweats, poultice or dirt and debris.

4. Properly place the legging appliance on the leg and secure with the Velcro straps making sure the heating pads run parallel to the tendons.

5. Plug in the legging appliance again and leave on the low setting until the patient becomes acquainted with the therapy.

6. After a few minutes turn the setting to high.

7. After approximately 10-15 minutes, turn the setting on low for the duration of the treatment.

8 When the treatment is concluded, the inside of the leggings should be wiped down with a mild disinfectant, dried and stored in a clean place.

9 A rigorous massage to the tendons and ligaments after therapy is ideal.

Due to the unique technology employed with the Thermotex™ Infrared Therapy System leggings, overheating of the tissues will not occur. When warming the legs before an event, a short duration of treatment is indicated but when therapy is initiated as a treatment for a clinical condition, long treatment times are very beneficial.

General Guidelines For Use with the Thermotex™ Infrared Therapy System Neck Appliance:

The average equine head weighs approximately 80 pounds. The support of this anatomical structure lies totally on the neck. Infrared heat therapy applied to this cervical *musculature* provides a relief of soreness and a more relaxed positioning of the head.

The following steps should be followed when applying the Thermotex™ Infrared Therapy System neck appliance:

1 Before the initiation of therapy, make sure the animal is properly restrained by either tying up the head or placing the animal in cross-ties.

2 Insure that the neck area is clean and free of all topical applications of any medications, liniments or sweats.

3 Preheat the neck appliance by plugging in and letting it warm on the high setting for a few minutes.

4 Properly place the appliance on the animal and secure with either the straps or use a soft cotton leg wrap.

The Thermotex™ Infrared Therapy neck appliance in use.

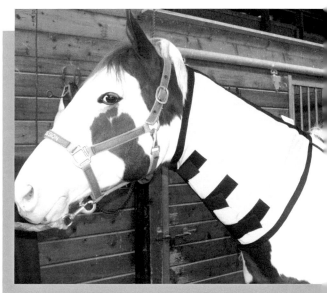

Chapter 2

5 Plug in the neck appliance and make sure the cords are out of reach of the animal's mouth and feet.

6 Turn the setting on high for at least the first 10 – 15 minutes of therapy.

7 The remainder of the determined therapy can be accomplished at the low setting on the control switch.

8 After the therapy is finished, clean the inside of the neck appliance with a mild disinfectant, dry and store in a clean place.

9 A thorough massage using both light and deep techniques is ideal after using the Thermotex™ Infrared Therapy System neck appliance.

Guidelines For Using the Thermotex™ Infrared Therapy System Hood Appliances:

The two hood appliances each allow for the topical application of infrared heat therapy. There are two models of hoods to choose from. The Therapeutic hood has a 3-inch wide by 8 inch long pad that fits directly over the frontal *sinuses* of the head and the same size pad that fits directly upon the ventral portion of the throat. The TMJ hood is designed with two heat elements that are directly over the TMJ of the horse and has two elements over the muscles of the upper part of the neck.

The following general guidelines will allow maximum utilization of these devices:

1 Secure the patient's head by tying it up or placing the animal in cross-ties.

2 Brush any dirt from the head and loosen the halter one or two notches.

3 Pre-warm the appliance by plugging it in and placing it on the high setting for a few minutes.

4 Fasten the hood comfortably on the patient using the Velcro straps.

5 Turn the switch to the high setting for the initial ten minutes of therapy.

6 Watch the animal closely for any signs of fear or discomfort from the hood being too snug.

7 After the initial ten minutes, turn the heat to the low setting and maintain this setting until the therapy session is completed.

8 Disinfect the inside of the hood after use and allow to dry before storage.

9 If necessary, sponge off the animal's head after treatment.

Conclusions:

Only our imagination and ingenuity limit the many uses of the Thermotex™ Infrared Therapy Systems products. Each animal is unique and requires its own tailored therapy program. Common sense, horsemanship and cleanliness are the basic foundation in the myriad of uses these products are capable of performing.

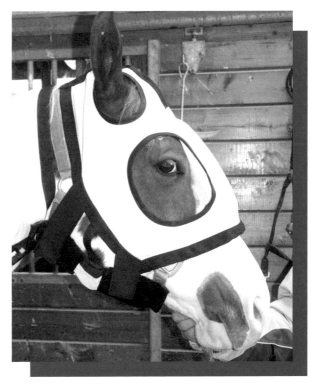

The Thermotex™ Infrared Therapy hood in use.

Chapter 2

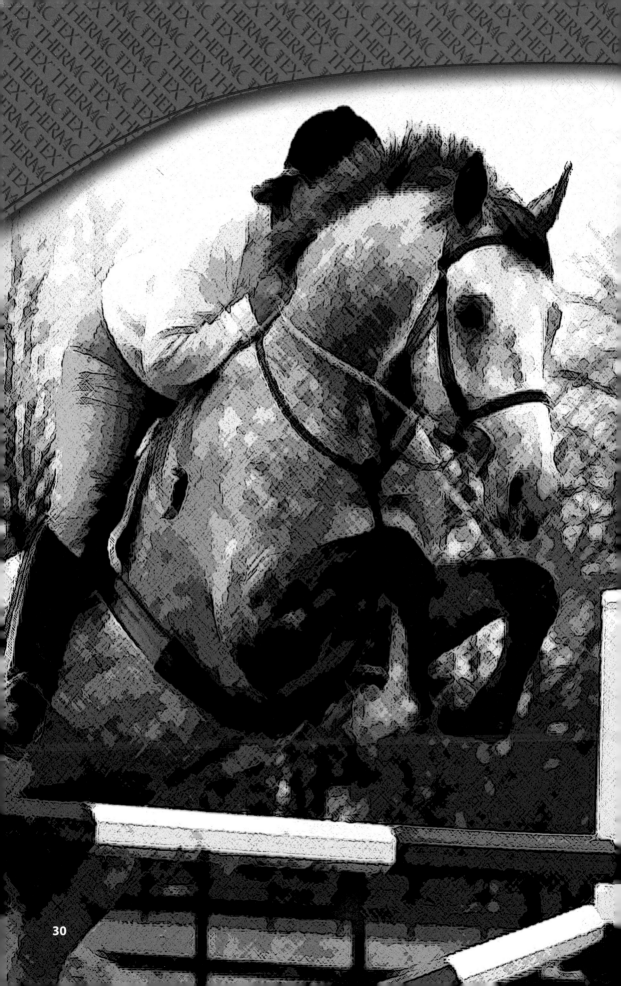

CHAPTER THREE

Therapy Protocols Using the Thermotex™ ITS Twelve Element Blanket

Introduction:

Whether your goal is clinical treatment of a disorder, an accelerated warm-up for an event, routine maintenance and prevention of problems or as an adjunct to other physical therapy modalities such as massage, the twelve element Thermotex™ Infrared Therapy Systems Blanket is the best topical heat producing physical therapy modality on the market. Once you start using this blanket, the many uses you will find for this infrared device will benefit your horse immensely.

Pre-Event Warm-Up:

Most equine athletes require a large amount of time to properly warm-up before their respective athletic discipline. Traditionally, this warm-up period starts out at a walk and then proceeds to light exercise as the animal becomes more limber and supple. The goal of this warm-up period is to increase the circulation, increase the tendon and ligament extensibility and decrease stiffness. These are all functions of what the Thermotex™ Infrared Therapy Systems Blanket accomplishes while the animal is still in the cross-ties.

> **Did you know?**
>
> *Human studies on Olympic athletes have revealed pre-event warm-up protocols have increased individual athletic ability by 10-12%.*

Using the average Hunter/Jumper as an example, the following traditional warm-up is used almost universally:

- The animal is removed from its stall and cleaned.
- A series of stretching exercises are undertaken depending on the age and condition of the animal.

- The animal is tacked and the rider mounts.
- The rider walks the animal for at least ten minutes or until the trainer deems the animal loose.
- A light trot is initiated for at least another fifteen minutes before the animal is galloped at any speed.
- This heavy work continues for another ten minutes or until the animal is completely warmed up and ready to jump.
- At this point, the real training begins whether it focuses on lead changes, jumping or merely equitation and approaches to the jumps. This phase can last anywhere from at least 30 minutes to an hour depending on the level of the horse.

Using this traditional regime the average total time it takes to get this animal ready to perform is 25 to 35 minutes. This is a hypothetical animal. A gifted young horse would require a shorter amount of time and yet an even longer amount of time would be required for an aged campaigner.

Utilizing the Thermotex™ Infrared Therapy Systems Blanket will save at least fifteen minutes of this time and allow the animal to perform more efficiently and comfortably when asked. If there are eight animals to train that day, this is a total savings of two hours in time that could be better spent in actually working and teaching the animal to perform at a higher level.

This new more efficient approach is as follows:

- Remove the animal from the stall; place in the cross-ties and clean.
- Properly fit the Thermotex™ Infrared Therapy Systems Blanket upon the animal after giving it a few minutes to warm up while you brush the horse.
- Turn the blanket on high for at least ten minutes and then lower it to the low setting for at least another twenty minutes. This therapy can be done while you are completing other chores or training another horse.
- Remove the blanket and properly take care of it.
- Give the animal a light massage and go through the stretching routine.
- Tack the animal, mount and ride.
- After only a few minutes of walking, you will be able to trot. After five minutes of this you will be able to extend the trot and start a heavier workload.

Now let's take this same animal to a jumping show where time is really tight and you want the maximum performance out of each animal. The following protocol could be followed to achieve the best athletic performance possible:

- Remove the animal from the stall; place in the cross-ties and clean.
- Properly fit the Thermotex™ Infrared Therapy Systems Blanket upon the animal after giving it a few minutes to warm up while you brush the horse.
- Turn the blanket on high for at least ten minutes and then lower it to the low setting for at least another twenty minutes.
- Tack and exercise the animal until completely warm.
- Place the animal back in the cross-ties and remove the tack. Again place the Thermotex™ Infrared Therapy Systems Blanket on the animal and turn it onto the low setting. Meanwhile, you can change into your show clothes while an attendant keeps an eye on your horse.

This sequence can be repeated several times throughout the day depending on the number of classes you have.

Standardbred example:

The faster the Standardbred or the older the Standardbred, the more they will benefit from the use of the Thermotex™ Infrared Therapy Systems Blanket. For these animals to perform at the highest efficiency possible and at the highest speed, they must be properly warmed up and pain free.

Traditionally, the standardbred racehorse is trained by jogging on the track in the wrong direction for a few miles and then turned and asked for speed. By using the Thermotex™ Infrared Therapy Systems Blanket on the equine athlete before the animal ever reaches the track, they step onto the track already relaxed, more supple and a more efficient and comfortable athlete. This allows a maximum performance and effort during each training session.

The following protocol is typical of a training day regimen:

- The horse is removed from the stall, placed in the cross-ties and cleaned.
- The Thermotex™ Infrared Therapy Systems Blanket is pre-warmed and placed on the animal for ten minutes at the high setting.

> " Another satisfied customer is Larry Jones. Larry is one of the best trainers on the Iowa and Kentucky circuit. He uses his two Thermotex™ blankets with excellent results. His Filly, Island Sands, came in second in the Kentucky Oaks and won the Acorn at Belmont. "
> – John Michaluk

- An additional twenty minutes of therapy is then initiated at the low setting.
- The blanket is removed and the animal is harnessed.

You will find that just after a mile of jogging, this animal is ready to train. Therefore, one not only saves time but also the animal endures less pounding on the track.

On race day there is a similar treatment protocol that can be followed:

- The animal can be warmed up in the stable with the use of the blanket before it ever hits the track.
- Depending on the animal's individual needs, the animal can be taken on the track and then turned for a brief lap approximately 40 to 60 minutes before its race.
- Upon returning to the stable, the animal is then treated again with the blanket allowing the animal to stay warm and not cool down before the race.
- Remove the blanket and then warm up normally just before the start of the race.

It doesn't really matter what discipline the equine athlete is utilized for; be it polo to dressage, show jumping to racing or even barrels to western pleasure. There is not one athletic event that would not benefit from a pre-event warm-up with the Thermotex™ Infrared Therapy Systems Blanket.

Any horse in any athletic event will benefit from a pre-event warm-up with the Thermotex™ blanket

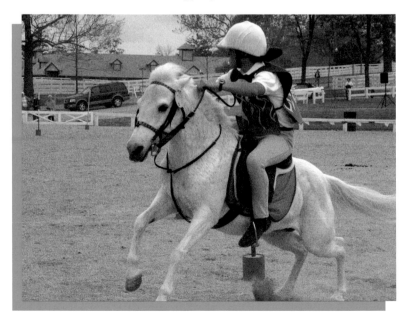

Treatment of Clinical Disorders Utilizing the Thermotex™ Infrared Therapy Systems Blanket:

Several equine clinical disorders benefit greatly from the use of the Thermotex™ Infrared Therapy Systems Blanket. These are but not limited to:

Myositis

Exertional Rhabdomyolysis (tying up)

Various neurological disorders

Secondary compensatory lameness

Myositis:

The term myositis can simply be broken down to reveal its meaning with "myo" meaning muscle and "itis" meaning an *inflammation* thereof. This inflammation can originate from trauma, bacteria, viruses or even through the administration of irritating substances through injections.

The inflammatory response within muscle tissue is a series of sequenced events that occurs after any insult to the muscle. Immediately after a traumatic insult to the muscle tissues, there is a brief constriction of blood vessels that lasts for just a few milliseconds. Then the blood vessels dilate to allow an increased blood flow. The injured muscle tissues release *histamine*, serotonin, and kinins. All of these result in a *vasodilatation* and an increased permeability within the walls of the blood vessels. The tissue swells and this is referred to as edema. Pain is also elicited within the area because of the presence of toxic substances on the sensory nerve endings.

Initially, cold therapy is utilized to cause a vasoconstriction and a reduction in the swelling. However, within 24 hours, infrared heat therapy is uniquely beneficial. Infrared heat therapy will have the following beneficial effects upon this inflamed muscle tissue:

There will be an increase in circulation that will allow for more nutrients to be present to the healing muscle cells and an increased capacity to carry away the toxic byproducts of inflammation.

Edema will be reduced in most cases because of the increased blood flow allowing drainage to the area.

Pain will be reduced by the mechanisms mentioned and this will expedite a break in the inflammatory response.

If the myositis is localized to a small area, the application of a single Thermotex™ Infrared Therapy Systems Heating pad may be all the therapy required. A single pad can be removed from the blanket and placed directly over the insulting area for a period of at least 30 minutes.

Most cases of myositis, especially when they are bacterial or viral in nature, are more generalized and treatment of the entire animal is beneficial. Follow all of the steps in preparing the patient for treatment as outlined above. Be patient and kind to the animal. Remember they are sick and in pain. Place the blanket on the animal and set on the high setting for approximately five minutes. Switch the setting to low and continue treatment for at least another 30 minutes to one hour. Multiple treatments throughout the day are ideal with three or four being optimum.

Exertional Rhabdomyolysis:

This is a muscular disorder commonly referred to by owners and trainers as "Monday morning sickness," *azoturia*, "tying up," myositis or exertional myositis. This disorder can range from a mild stiffness of the *musculature* to actual cramping and recumbency. The initial stiffness usually occurs in the neck muscles and over the gluteal areas. These animals will sweat excessively and have elevated cardiovascular and respiratory rates in addition to a slight increase in body temperature. When the muscles are palpated, there is pain elicited with only minor digital pressure. The muscles feel tense and stiff, especially along the longissimus dorsi and gluteal regions. Another classic symptom of these horses is a *myoglobinuria*, which horsemen refer to as coffee-colored urine.

This muscular disorder occurs when an animal is rested for a period of time during a training program and then returned to hard work. The nickname "Monday morning sickness" was coined when this disorder was first seen in draft animals used six days a week, rested on Sunday, and returned to hard work on Monday morning. These animals would then exhibit rhabdomyolysis on Mondays. Endurance horses that are improperly trained will usually exhibit this myopathy after the first day of an event.

The *etiology* of exertional rhabdomyolysis is not clearly understood. A change in the blood supply within the muscle tissue, a fluid and/or electrolyte imbalance, a genetic predisposition, or a nutritional influence have all been indicated in causing exertional rhabdomyolysis.

The only clinical sign that one would notice in a mild case is a slight change in the gait or merely that an animal is performing at a lower level than expected. There may be pain and stiffness upon palpation of the neck or gluteal musculature. An elevated heart rate and respiratory rate may be evident. In severe cases, the horse may exhibit extreme pain, a reluctance to move, severe stiffness and sweating. It is in this stage that the animal usually exhibits a myoglobinuria. Occasionally, these animals are in a state of recumbency.

Treatment of these animals should be focused on ***analgesia***, a reduction in further muscle damage and the restoration of fluid and electrolyte balances.

Infrared heat therapy using the Thermotex™ Infrared Therapy Systems Blanket has greatly reduced the inflammation within the muscles and greatly reduced the recovery time of these animals. In severe cases it is often advantageous to seek veterinary assistance to help with the pain management and fluid therapy. These treatments coupled with the therapy that the Thermotex™ Infrared Therapy Systems Blanket insures a speedy recovery and a return to athletic competition.

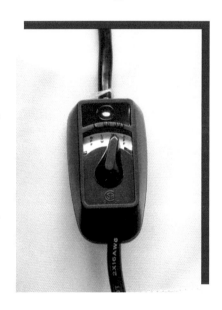

The Thermotex™ control has high and low settings for different applications.

The following guidelines will aid in the treatment of this condition:

Acute:

Immediately upon diagnosis of exertional rhabdomyolysis place the pre-warmed Thermotex™ Infrared Therapy Systems Blanket on the patient at the low setting. This can be accomplished while other treatments such as fluid therapy are initiated.

The high setting can be used when the animal is in extreme discomfort. Ten to fifteen minutes on the high setting is sufficient to achieve a deeper penetration of the heat and a higher level of relaxation and analgesia. After this time the switch should be again placed on the low setting.

Keep the blanket on the animal until the recovery is complete. Simply unplug it when therapy is not required and place other blankets on top of it if needed for warmth.

Therapy sessions should be long and often throughout the day. The more therapy, the quicker the recovery.

Chronic:

Before each exercise session, these animals should be warmed up using the Thermotex™ Infrared Therapy Systems Blanket for at least thirty minutes.

After warm-up and stretching their exercise session should begin and then end with a long cool down period.

Later in the day, after the animal has been properly cooled down and cared for, a second therapy session should be initiated to increase the blood flow and rid the muscles of any lactic acid and other metabolic byproducts produced by the morning's workout. This session should last approximately thirty minutes.

Prevention of another acute episode is the goal of therapy to these animals and one can't use the Thermotex™ Infrared Therapy Systems Blanket enough. There is no danger in overheating the patient or causing any dehydration through the use of this appliance, therefore one can't overuse the product.

Neurological Disorders:

Almost all neurological disorders have some effect upon the musculature. These effects range from muscle atrophy in severe cases to slight dysfunction that appears as a mild form of undetermined lameness. Any disorder that has a direct effect upon the musculature can benefit from the Thermotex™ Infrared Therapy Systems Blanket.

Three of the most common neurological disorders affecting the musculature are equine herpesvirus myeloencephalopathy, hyperkalemic periodic paralysis and equine protozoal myeloencephalitis. These are not the only neurological disorders of the horse but these are ones most commonly seen affecting the musculature.

Equine Herpesvirus Myeloencephalopathy

Whenever there is a large concentration of horses such as the racetrack, breeding farm or boarding stable, there is a high incidence of viral infections. Equine herpesvirus type 4 (EHV-4) is a major cause of respiratory tract disease in horses, whereas EHV-1 is the strain responsible for the myeloencephalopathy. This can occur in horses of all ages and has an incubation time of approximately seven days after initial exposure.

These animals develop a fever and there is usually evidence of a mild respiratory tract disorder. This may be manifested merely

> " Throughout years of involvement with high performance horses, I have found that Thermotex is a user friendly blanket that is beneficial for relaxation thereby allowing stiff joints to loosen and get blood flowing to the area. This enables my stretching routine to proceed without pain or injury. Regular use of the Thermotex blanket will result in a strong, steady, powerful, painfree, happy horse. Thermotex is a powerful tool. I swear by it. "
>
> – Julie Bridge
> Equine Yoga
> Calgary, Australia

as a cough or a slight nasal discharge. Initially, the animal may show signs of a slight lameness or abnormal gait. As the virus progresses, the animal may appear stiff and show signs of weakness and ataxia within the limbs.

After a diagnosis is made, supportive care using the Thermotex™ Infrared Therapy Systems Blanket can be initiated immediately concurrent with other treatment modalities. Several treatments a day will not only make the animal more comfortable but it will speed the recovery of the muscles from the effects of the virus. The following is a hypothetical treatment regime:

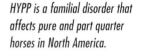
- Pre-warm the blanket for a few minutes on the high setting before placing on the patient.
- Place the blanket on the horse and turn the switch to the high setting for 10 minutes.
- After 10 minutes, lower the temperature to the low setting for the duration of the treatment.
- After 20 minutes, move the pads to a different position within their pockets; this allows more of the muscle group to be treated.
- The therapy session should last at least one hour in duration.
- Remove the blanket, sanitize, dry and store.
- Blanket the animal with a light sheet or blanket so that it does not become chilled.

HYPP is a familial disorder that affects pure and part quarter horses in North America.

Hyperkalemic Periodic Paralysis (HYPP):

This disorder involves the peripheral nerves and musculature. It is a familial disorder that affects pure and part quarter horses in North America. HYPP is similar to hyperkalemic periodic paralysis in people in that these animals undergo episodes of muscular weakness. It is more common in colts than in fillies, and it usually affects horses that are less than 4 years old.

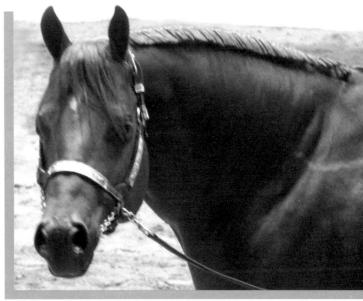

These animals are extremely well muscled and appear absolutely normal between episodes of weakness. Any stressful stimuli such as exercise, high environmental temperature or transport may precipitate a clinical manifestation of this disorder. Episodes of hyperkalemic periodic paralysis, however, may be totally unpredictable and occur at random. Initially, the animal will appear still and will have a prolapse of the third eyelid. The horse will begin to sweat, and muscle fasciculation will occur. As the episode progresses, these animals become recumbent and the muscles develop flaccidity. The horse's respiratory and heart rates are usually elevated. The animal will be alert and able to respond to noise and visual stimuli. These episodes usually last between 15 to 20 minutes.

Treatment consists of an intravenous administration of sodium bicarbonate, dextrose, potassium free isotonic fluids and insulin. Intravenous administration of calcium gluconate, diluted in a dextrose solution, at a rate of 40 – 90 mg/Kg usually results in a rapid remission of the clinical signs.

Following one of these episodes, the animal is usually quite stiff and muscle sore. A number of therapy sessions with the Thermotex™ Infrared Therapy Systems Blanket will speed the recovery and hasten the return to athletic competition. These episodes quite commonly occur at a horse show due to the added stress to these animals. A fast recovery is often the difference between a wasted trip and a successful event. The following guidelines have been used effectively to treat these animals with the Thermotex™ Infrared Therapy Systems Blanket at the horse show:

- After the diagnosis is made and the intravenous treatment has begun, the Thermotex™ Infrared Therapy Systems Blanket is placed on the animal.
- This blanket should be pre-heated and the switch should be on high initially for at least 15 minutes.
- Therapy should continue at the low setting for another hour or until the symptoms have dissipated.
- Unplug and leave the blanket on the animal and hand walk the animal when possible.
- Treat the animal every few hours with an initial high setting on the switch for approximately 10 minutes and then low for another long session.
- Be careful that the animal stays warm at all times.

You cannot over treat these animals with the Thermotex™ Infrared Therapy Systems Blanket. Several treatments in a 24-hour period will almost eliminate muscle soreness and any other side effects the episode had on the musculature.

Equine Protozoal Myeloencephalitis (EPM):

Equine protozoal myeloencephalitis is a debilitating disease of the horse that results in asymmetric incoordination, weakness, spasticity and may be potentially fatal. This disorder is caused by the protozoan *Sarcocytis falcatula*. This organism can affect horses of all ages but is more commonly diagnosed in horses less than four years of age.

Treatment of equine protozoal myeloencephalitis has the goals of eliminating the parasite, reducing the inflammation within the nervous tissue and treating any secondary complications. It is these secondary complications within the musculature where the Thermotex™ Infrared Therapy Systems Blanket is employed.

The nervous system becomes incapacitated in its ability to properly stimulate the muscle tissues. This results in a state of incoordination and ataxia. Once the diagnosis of EPM is made, infrared heat therapy to the musculature should be initiated. If caught in the early stages, recovery from the symptoms can usually be seen in three to four days. Therapy sessions should be performed using common sense and will be unique for each case. These simple guidelines offer a place to start:

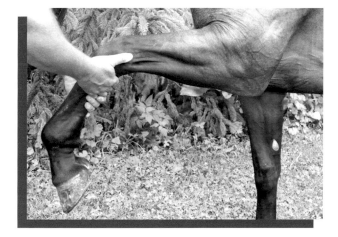

Thermotex™ Infrared Therapy is beneficial in treating the secondary complications associated with EPM.

- Initially, the patient will be merely foul gaited to one that is ataxic in nature. Therapy sessions should be performed a minimum of once per day to several times per day.

- In all cases, pre-warm the blanket and place it on the high setting for at least 15 minutes during the initial therapy.

- Since the goal is an increase in circulation within the musculature, long therapy sessions at the low temperature setting are ideal.

- After the therapy session is over, digital massage of the muscles will aid in their recovery.

Using the Thermotex™ Infrared Therapy Systems Blanket for the Treatment of Secondary Compensatory Lameness:

The equine athlete is a marvel of locomotor biomechanics. When a problem occurs within this biological machine, the entire organism is affected. Therefore, if a primary lameness problem occurs in the foot, all of the anatomical structures proximal to the foot are also affected. Offering the right hind foot as an example: there is a stone bruise on the inside of this foot. This affects the way the animal now lands on the foot which affects the stress on the ankle which affects the stress on the hock and stifle which ultimately affects the back of the horse in all of the muscles. This is how the horse compensates for a lameness problem. Therefore, don't fall into the habit of treating only the primary point of lameness in this case i.e. the stone bruise, treat all of the anatomical structures involved with this lameness (secondary lameness) and recovery will be expedited.

Any lower limb lameness will affect the musculature of the back.

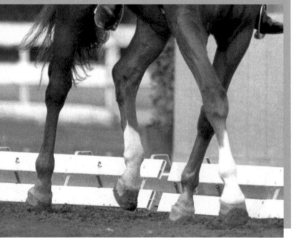

All lower limb lameness affects the musculature of the horse's back. Therefore, it is only logical to utilize the Thermotex™ Infrared Therapy Systems Blanket to alleviate any secondary soreness within these muscles. A normal therapy regimen should be followed at least once per day with more aggressive plans initiated if the lameness is more severe. These therapy sessions should last at least an hour to allow for the full physiological effects of the blanket to take place.

Utilization of the Thermotex™ Infrared Therapy Systems Blanket During the Training Regime For the Prevention of Muscle Soreness:

Using the Thermotex™ Infrared Therapy Systems Blanket as a daily routine therapy device greatly alleviates muscle soreness and pain to the equine athlete in training. Ideally, all of the horses in training should have the benefit of a pre-event warm-up before the initiation of the daily training program. After a particular rigorous training session or work at speed, it is very beneficial to undergo another therapy session later in the day after the animal has cooled out. The Thermotex™ Infrared Therapy Systems Blanket is so easy to use, effective and almost non-labor intensive that using it on a daily basis reaps many rewards.

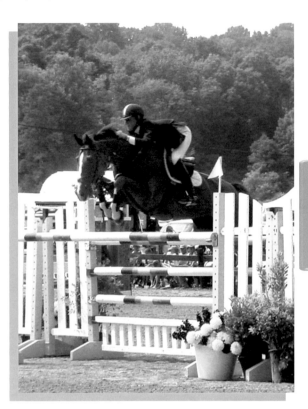

Regardless of the discipline, preparing the animal for the daily rigors of training will allow an efficient use of the time spent training the horse. Just like their human counterparts in athletic training, the daily wear and tear has both physical and psychological effects upon the athlete. Why not prepare the equine athlete to take that first training step more comfortable, more supple and therefore more efficient at using the time allotted for training?

A warm-up of just 30 minutes will allow the animal to be more comfortable by relieving the stiffness and soreness that occurs from a daily training program. Training a slightly lame or sore horse is frustrating and non-rewarding. This quick 30-minute treatment will allow you to train a horse that is relaxed and virtually pain free at the initiation of the training procedure.

Preparing the horse with a 30 minute Infrared warm-up session will help you make the most of your daily training program.

The axiom in every gym is "no pain; no gain." Our equine athletes have the same daily problems in training as the human athletes. Therefore, daily use of the Thermotex™ Infrared Therapy Systems Blanket will also have a psychological effect upon the equine athlete. When they are more comfortable they will be more willing to train and will train more efficiently.

Extra therapy sessions later in the day after the workout can only help the equine athlete. If there is a day during the week where the training is at a higher level than normal, it is advantageous to aid in the recovery from that training. After the animal has been cooled and properly taken care of, a second therapy session is extremely beneficial. This can be 30 minutes to 60 minutes in

Chapter 3

duration. After this second treatment, it is beneficial to walk the animal for at least 15 – 20 minutes with a light sheet to allow the muscles a light work. This will really speed the recovery from the rigorous workout earlier in the day.

Using the Thermotex™ Infrared Therapy Systems Blanket as Part of a Total Equine Therapy Program:

Massage Therapy:

The benefits of massage have been scientifically proven throughout the years. What better way to prepare a patient for massage than a pretreatment with the Thermotex™ Infrared Therapy Systems Blanket?

Beginning the massage therapy session with an animal that is already relaxed and supple allows a more thorough and efficient massage. Muscles that are stiff, sore and in a state of spasm at the onset of a routine massage are now supple, relaxed and more responsive to therapy. Normally, it takes 15 –20 minutes on the average to prepare the equine patient for deep fundamental massage work. By 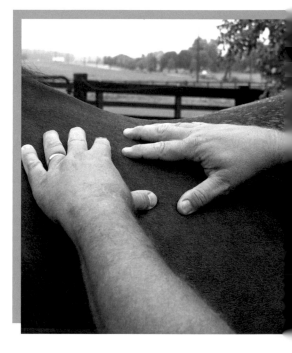 pre-warming the patient, the light effleurage and stroking portion of the therapy can be accomplished in about half of the time that it normally takes. This then allows more time for deep work on problem areas or more time stretching to restore full range of motion within the limbs.

Most barns have more than one horse receiving massage therapy at a given time. Start the initial animal with a 30-minute therapy session while you gather history and maintain your records for the animals. Remove the blanket from this animal and place it on the second animal while you are massaging the first. This gives this animal an extra hour of therapy before you even begin the massage! This second animal will be a very willing patient and will get the maximum effect from the massage. When the second animal is massaged, move the blanket to the third animal and progress in this fashion until all of the animals receiving therapy that day have been treated.

Chiropractic Manipulation:

The philosophy behind chiropractic care is based on the relationship of the spinal column to the nervous system and the role of the spinal column in the fundamental biomechanics of locomotion.

The equine athlete benefits greatly from chiropractic manipulations. Peak athletic performance can only be achieved when the athlete is free of soreness, stiffness and pain. To put this in perspective: if a human sprinter has sore lower back muscles, how well will they perform? All of the major muscles of locomotion are attached to the highly jointed vertebral column. This structure is highly important to the performance of the athletic animal.

Use of the Thermotex™ Infrared Therapy Systems Blanket upon the major muscles of the back allows for a more relaxed, supple chiropractic patient. The twelve-element blanket contains a series of infrared heat pads that follow the musculature in close proximity on both sides of the spine. This deep penetrating heat results in relaxation, analgesia and an increased blood flow to this area. This ultimately allows for more efficient chiropractic manipulation and adjustment.

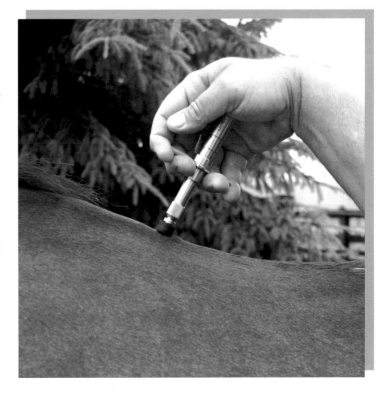

The longer the blanket is on a patient, the more beneficial the therapy. Warming the patient in the blanket for at least a 30-minute session will allow an easier chiropractic manipulation. Use the normal therapy protocol of placing the blanket on the high setting for at least 10 – 15 minutes and then on low for the duration of the therapy. When treating an animal with a great deal of soreness throughout the spinal musculature, therapy sessions with the Thermotex™ Infrared Therapy Systems Blanket can be up to an hour in length. Many times it is beneficial to the patient to repeat these infrared heat treatments multiple times during the day.

Other Uses of the Thermotex™ Infrared Therapy Systems Blanket:

Only our intelligence limits us to the potential usefulness of this product. Over the years the blanket has been used in the following unique situations:

- As a field incubator for neonatal foal intensive care.
- As an aid in the treatment of shock.
- Adjunct therapy to an animal suffering an allergic reaction.
- Numerous cases of trauma.
- To help ease the spasms of Tetanus.
- As an aid in the recovery of the musculature from a patient who suffered seizures.
- To comfort mares suffering from Hypocalcemia.
- To increase the blood supply to various lacerations to speed the healing process.
- Aid in the recovery of "Sweeny."
- As an aid to speed the healing process on various abscesses.
- Acute laminitis.
- As an aid in the recovery from an epileptic seizure.

Conclusions:

The uses for this unique equine physical therapy device are almost infinite. To quote Hippocrates: "Above All, Do No Harm." With the Thermotex™ Infrared Therapy Systems Blanket one need not worry about doing any harm. Overheating or burning of the patient is not a concern. All of the patients who receive therapy from this appliance will experience muscle relaxation, relief from pain and a decrease in soreness and stiffness. The final result of this is that they will reach their full athletic potential.

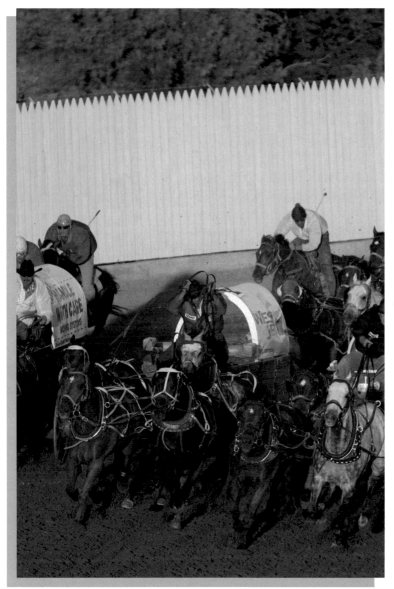

Horses in any discipline will benefit from infrared therapy.

Racing chuck wagons photo courtesy of the Calgary Stampede.

Visit their website at www.calgarystampede.com for more information

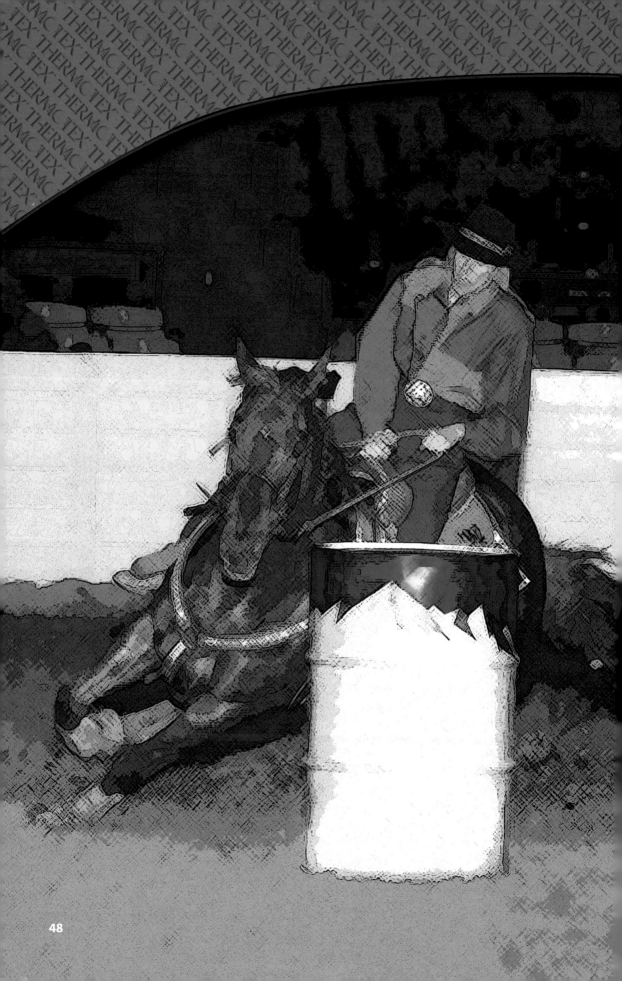

CHAPTER FOUR

Basic Therapeutic Treatment Protocols Using the Thermotex™ ITS Extended Leggings

Introduction:

The Thermotex™ Infrared Therapy System Leggings are a hinged, well-designed infrared heating appliance that can be used on either the forelimbs or hind. Each legging contains four heating elements encased in the same easy care material that the therapy blanket is made of. Each Leggings unit is supplied in pairs so that either front or hind limbs can be treated simultaneously.

If a clinical problem exists, consult a veterinarian before treatment is initiated. An example of this concern can be illustrated by a simple swelling within the flexor tendons of the lower limb. One should ask why these tissues are swollen and an immediate accurate diagnosis should be made before any type of therapy is initiated.

The following physiological effects are the result of the application of infrared therapeutic heat to the lower limbs of the horse:

- *Vasodilatation* and increased blood flow throughout all of the tissues.

- *Analgesia*.

- Increased extensibility within the ligaments and tendons.

- Decrease in joint stiffness.

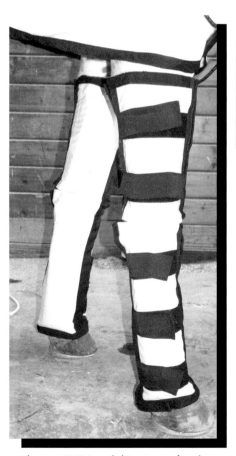

Thermotex™ ITS Extended Leggings on front legs.

Chapter 4

Basic Therapeutic Treatment Protocols Using the Thermotex™ ITS Extended Leggings   **49**

To achieve these desired physiological effects, the application of infrared therapeutic heat and the duration of treatment should be consistent with your goals of therapy.

Equipment and Patient Basics When Using the Thermotex™ Infrared Therapy System Leggings:

The following general step-by-step guidelines should be considered when applying this unique modality to the lower limbs:

1. The horse should have its head tied up or be placed in a set of cross-ties. In some cases a muzzle will need to be utilized.

2. All dirt, poultice, liniments or any topically applied substances should be removed from the limb either by brushing or with a hose and water.

3. Pre-warm the leggings by plugging them in and placing them on high for a few minutes.

4. Place the leggings on the desired limb or limbs and secure with the Velcro straps. Patience must be exercised when attempting this for the first time, as this is a strange concept for the horse to understand.

5. Make sure the legging appliance and all electric cords are out of reach of the animals' mouth and feet.

6. Turn the switch to the low setting initially until the animal becomes acquainted with the therapy. After a few minutes, set the switch to high for at least 10 - 15 minutes.

7. Continue the therapy at the low setting for the duration of the treatment.

8. When the treatment is concluded, the inside of the leggings should be wiped down with a mild disinfectant, dried and stored in a clean place.

9. A rigorous massage to the tendons and ligaments after therapy is ideal.

Therapy times will vary depending upon the goal. If the leggings are used as a pre-event warm-up of the ligaments and tendons before exercise, the therapy should last approximately 30 minutes. If the goal of therapy is to treat a clinical condition, then longer and multiple treatments are beneficial.

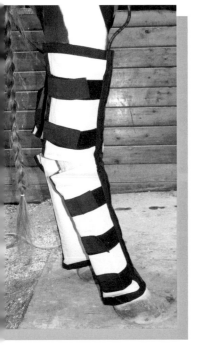

Thermotex™ ITS Extended Leggings on hind legs.

Using the Thermotex™ Infrared Therapy System Leggings as a Pre-Event Warm-Up:

By using the Thermotex™ Infrared Therapy System Leggings before exercising, the animal takes that first step out of the barn more comfortable and flexible. Both the tendons and ligaments within the limb are more extensible which allows a greater range of motion within the limb. This allows the animal to start an exercise program 10 to 15 minutes ahead of schedule.

Using the leggings upon joints such as the knee, ankle and hock allows the ligamentous and tendonous structures around these joints to be more flexible and extensible. There will be a decrease in the *viscosity* of the *synovial* fluid within the joint. This will result in a more lubricated joint and a decrease in joint stiffness. The entire structure of the joint will experience a relief from pain due to sensory nerves recognizing heat messages and ignoring the pain messages. These factors all result in a joint that experiences a reduction in pain and has a greater range of motion. However, it should be noted that this therapy will relieve the symptoms of stiffness and increase the range of motion but will not cause a remission of a condition such as arthritis or degenerative joint disease.

Pre-event warm-up or pre-exercise warm-up benefits the horse regardless of its athletic endeavor or age. An aged racehorse or jumper will experience flexibility and pain relief before even starting their daily exercise program or competing in their event. Young animals in training are offered relief from their daily rigorous training and are therefore more willing to perform as well as perform at a higher level. Injuries to the tendons are less likely to happen since all of the soft tissue structures are more flexible.

> ## Teaching Tip
>
> Be patient when applying this appliance for the first time. Many animals find these leggings confining and slightly constricting, but patience will prevail.

Chapter 4

Using the Thermotex™ ITS Leggings as a Treatment for Common Lameness Disorders:

Forelimb Disorders:

Common Carpal (Knee) Disorders: The equine athlete places a tremendous amount of concussive forces upon the knee during heavy exercise. This results in *carpitis, carpal tunnel syndrome* and *degenerative joint disease* within the joints. The amount of concussive force placed upon this anatomical structure is a function of both the animal's conformation and its athletic event.

An overextension of the carpus, such as that when a cross country eventer clears a jump and the opposite side is sloped away from the jump, results in carpitis. Simply defined, *carpitis* is an inflammation within the tissues of the knee. This inflammation results in *osteitis*, inflammation of the bones, *periostitis* and pain within these structures.

Carpal tunnel syndrome results from an inflammation and pressure within the carpal canal usually caused by a *tendonitis* of the flexor tendons, a *desmitis* of the superior check ligament or a fracture in this area. As these tissues swell, pressure is applied upon the neurovascular supply to this area which results in a compensated blood flow to the distal tissues. This pressure also results in pain to the affected limb.

Degenerative joint disease of the carpus can be mild in nature to severely debilitating. Repetitive concussive trauma to the joints within the knee results in a thickening and fibrosis of the synovial membrane and joint capsule, a breakdown of the cartilage and a subsequent formation of *osteophytes* on the bony structures. These pathological changes result in a decrease in the ability of the joint to flex through its normal range of motion.

Repetitive concussive trauma can lead to degenerative joint disease.

Once an accurate diagnosis is made and a treatment plan is initiated, the application of infrared heat is a convenient modality to reduce swelling, alleviate pain and allow a greater elasticity within the tendons and ligaments. The end result of this application of heat is a restoration of the range of motion within the knee. General guidelines are as follows:

At least one hour before exercising, conduct a therapy session using the Thermotex™ Infrared Therapy System Leggings for at least 30 minutes upon both knees. After this is completed, take the limbs through normal range of motion stretches.

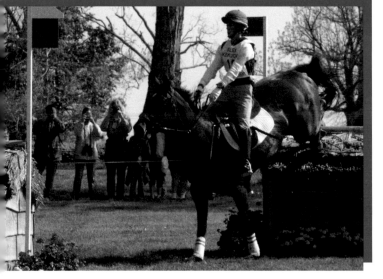

If infrared heat therapy is part of the treatment regime for a specific lameness disorder of the carpus, long therapy sessions at the low setting several times per day would be beneficial.

Immediately after a strenuous exercise or event it might be advantageous to first apply cold hydrotherapy to the knees, allow drying and then conduct a therapy session about 30 – 45 minutes in duration.

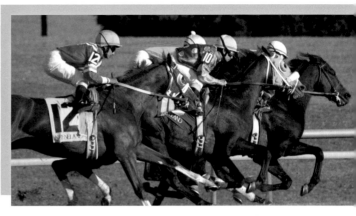

Soft tissue injuries of the forelimb are common in race horses.

Common Soft Tissue Disorders of the Forelimb:

Dorsal metacarpal disease ("Bucked Shins"), ***desmitis of the suspensory ligament, tendonitis, tendosynovitis, bowed tendons*** and ***inferior check ligament desmitis*** all can benefit from infrared heat therapy provided by the Thermotex™ Infrared Therapy System Leggings.

Horsemen traditionally refer to the slight inflammation and swelling on the dorsal surface of the third metacarpal bone as "bucked shins." The repetitive concussive trauma from the foot hitting the ground causes an inflammation within the ***periosteum*** (covering directly on the bone) and a remodeling of the dorsal cortex of the third metacarpal. If this remodeling cannot keep up with the trauma from the concussive forces, microfractures of this bony tissue will result.

At the first indication of swelling or pain, an accurate diagnosis should be made. If caught in the early stages, systemic anti-inflammatory and an intense physical therapy regime should be undertaken.

Many physical therapy modalities are effective in the treatment of this disorder. The goal of them all is to reduce the inflammation and pain while allowing the bone to remodel subsequent to the workload. Initially, cold therapy is indicated until the swelling and inflammatory process is stopped. After this is accomplished, alternate cold and therapeutic heat is indicated. A hypothetical therapy program is as follows:

- Cold therapy until the inflammation is gone.
- Alternating cold and therapeutic heat therapy until the animal is ready to begin exercise.
- A pre-exercise warm-up with the Thermotex™ ITS Leggings for at least 30 minutes before exercise.

Chapter 4

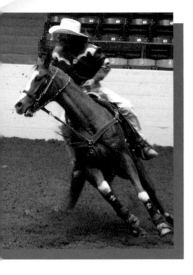

- Immediately after exercise, an application of cold therapy to halt any inflammation and subsequent microhemorrhages.
- Later in the day, a second therapeutic heat session for at least 30 minutes.

Any inflammation within the suspensory ligament is referred to as being a ***desmitis***. Usually there is a slight swelling within this structure and often a mild lameness. When palpated digitally, there is evidence of pain. When the condition is chronic, digital palpation will reveal scar tissue present.

When this injury is acute, cold therapy is the first measure to be taken. After 24 hours, alternating cold with infrared heat therapy will speed the healing process. An example of this regime is as follows:

- Apply cold therapy for 30 – 40 minutes, rest for two hours and then repeat.
- After the inflammation is under control, apply cold therapy for 30 minutes, rest for two hours, apply therapeutic infrared heat for 30 minutes on the low setting, rest for two hours, cold therapy for 30 minutes, rest for two hours, apply therapeutic infrared heat for 30 minutes on the low setting, etc.
- When the animal is ready to begin exercising again, apply infrared therapeutic heat for 30 minutes, exercise, apply cold therapy for 30 minutes, rest for two hours, apply infrared therapeutic heat for 30 minutes, rest for two hours, etc.

As the amount of exercise is increased, it may be necessary to increase the length of the therapy times and the frequency.

Tendonitis is simply any inflammation within the tendon. ***Tendosynovitis*** is any inflammation within the tendon sheath. Horsemen refer to any swelling or inflammation within the flexor tendons on the palmar aspect of the metacarpals as a ***"bowed tendon."*** Depending on their location, they are further classified as "high," "middle" and "low" bows. All of these pathological changes are the result of stress, strain and concussive force upon these anatomical structures.

Prevention of these disorders is the key to a sound training program. Regardless of the discipline, pre-exercise warm-up with the Thermotex™ Infrared Therapy System Leggings will aid in the prevention of these types of injuries. Therapy sessions of at least 30 minutes duration should be conducted before the exercise session. This will increase the blood flow to the tissues, make the tendons more flexible and provide a relief to existing soreness.

When these injuries have already occurred, and are in the acute stage, an aggressive physical therapy program should be initiated possibly using several different modalities. A hypothetical example of this type of program is as follows:

- In the acute stage, an application of cold therapy for at least 30 – 45 minutes several times per day. Ideally, this can be performed every two hours.

Did you know?

In the acute stage of an injury, apply cold therapy first and then alternate cold therapy with infrared therapeutic heat.

- After the inflammatory reaction is stemmed, alternating cold therapy with therapeutic heat will speed the healing process. If possible, cold therapy for 30 minutes, massage and rest for two hours, therapeutic heat for 30 minutes, massage and easy stretching, rest for two hours, cold therapy for 30 minutes, rest and light massage, therapeutic heat for 30 minutes, etc.
- When the animal is able to begin exercise, it is important to warm the tissues for at least 30 minutes prior to the exercise session. This will allow a reduction in the swelling and more flexible soft tissues. Immediately after exercise, cold therapy should be applied to halt any inflammation initiated by the exercise. After a period of rest, another therapeutic heat session should be conducted.

These steps are repeated and modified on an individual case basis until the animal is completely recovered from the injury. Exercising these animals in the future should always include a session of pre-event warm-up before stress to these soft tissues.

Desmitis of the inferior check ligament is a common disorder in trotters and pacers. Stress on this ligament occurs when an animal is shod with a long toe and low heal to obtain a longer stride. This coupled with an imbalanced situation towards the medial side of the foot results in a significant strain to this ligament.

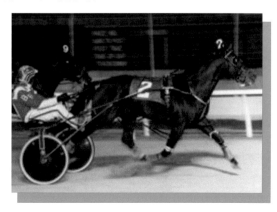

In the acute stage, cold therapy is indicated to reduce inflammation and swelling. This can then be followed by alternating cold and therapeutic heat until the problem is resolved.

Unfortunately, due to the conformation of the horse, this nagging injury becomes chronic. In these situations it is always advantageous to warm this tissue before exercise and then follow the exercise with cold therapy. There is no easier and safer way to warm these tissues than using the Thermotex™ Infrared Therapy System Leggings. Especially in a large stable where numerous animals are trained each day, the only efficient way to provide therapeutic heat for 30 minutes before exercise is with this modality.

The Thermotex™ Infrared Therapy System Leggings reach to the coronary band of the foot. This allows the application of therapeutic infrared heat to both the fetlock and pastern. Disorders such as *sesamoiditis, osselets, osteochondrosis* and *degenerative joint disease of the fetlock joint* and *ringbone* can be addressed using this physical therapy modality.

Constant repetitive concussive forces result in a stress and strain to the proximal sesamoid bones and their associated ligamentous structures. This in turn causes an inflammatory reaction within these tissues termed *sesamoiditis*.

These animals exhibit a mild lameness and exhibit pain upon digital palpation. Rest and corrective shoeing help alleviate this condition but they will recover faster with an aggressive physical therapy program.

In the acute stage, cold therapy is very beneficial for the first 24 to 48 hours. After this time, alternating cold and infrared therapeutic heat will speed the healing process. After recovery, pre-exercise warming of these tissues helps prevent reinjury.

Osselets are a traumatic arthritis of the metacarpophalangeal joint. This results from a capsulitis and synovitis at the dorsal aspect of the metacarpophalangeal joint. When these cases become chronic, there is an ossification that will develop within this capsule.

This condition results from athletic competition and training where there is a constant concussive trauma to the fetlock joint. When this disorder is in the acute stage, it is referred to

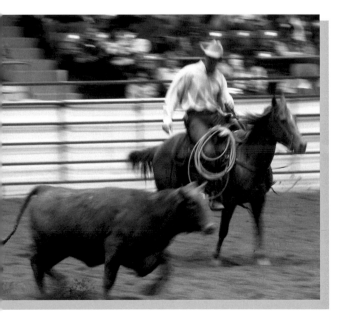

as a *"green osselet."* There is swelling and pain along the dorsal aspect of the fetlock. When the condition progresses, there will be a thickening within the joint capsule.

Aggressive physical therapy techniques coupled with systemic treatment, corrective shoeing and a change in the training program will greatly aid in the management of this disorder.

The following protocol will aid in the physical therapy management of these cases:

- In the acute stage, cold therapy is utilized until the inflammatory response is stopped. This usually takes multiple treatments, i.e. every two hours, over a 24-hour period.
- After 24 hours, alternate infrared therapeutic heat with cold therapy throughout the day.
- When exercise is initiated, pre-warm the tissues with an infrared heat therapy session. Immediately after exercise, cold therapy is applied for at least 30 minutes, followed by rest, followed by another session of infrared therapeutic heat.
- When the animal has recovered, always pre-warm the tissues before exercise with a 30-minute session of therapeutic infrared heat.

Osteochondrosis of the fetlock arises from genetic predisposition, rapid growth rates and nutritional imbalances. It is simply cartilage that fails to develop into healthy solid bony tissue. These areas are therefore weak and easily injured from the trauma of normal athletic activity.

There are two basic categories of osteochondrosis within the fetlock. Concussive trauma from athletic exercise results in these weakened areas to form subchondral bone cysts whereas shearing forces applied to these weakened areas result in a flap of cartilage within the joint itself. This flap or fragment of cartilage covering the chondro-osseous interface is referred to as an *osteochondritis dissecans lesion* or *OCD*.

These animals often exhibit an intermittent lameness or are very lame. There is swelling within the joint and pain upon flexion. An accurate diagnosis is made using radiographic techniques. Treatment regimes include: rest, intraarticular medications, systemic medications, arthroscopic surgery and aggressive physical therapy programs.

In mild early-diagnosed cases, rest coupled with physical therapy may allow this disorder to heal. Cold therapy is used for the first 24 hours to alleviate swelling and break the

> ### Teaching Tip
>
> Only a thorough radiographic study will reveal OCD lesions. Regardless of the treatment protocol, aggressive physical therapy with infrared heat will expedite the recovery time.

Chapter 4

inflammatory cycle. After this period of time, alternate cold and infrared heat therapy is used to speed the recovery period.

Maintenance of these animals should always include infrared heat therapy. Before any exercise, pre-event warm-up procedures should be undertaken for a minimum of 30 minutes.

If arthroscopic surgery is indicated, recovery from this procedure can be accelerated through the use of infrared therapeutic heat. Just a few days after surgery, infrared heat sessions should be conducted along with guidance from the attending surgeon.

Ringbone is new bone growth that originates and forms on the dorsal, dorsolateral, and dorsomedial surfaces of the first and second phalanges and the extensor process of the third phalanx. There are four forms of ringbone: high, low, periarticular and articular.

Ringbone is caused by concussive trauma to the tissues. Conformationally challenged animals are predisposed to this disorder when they are asked to perform at a high level within their athletic discipline.

If this disorder is detected in the early stages, aggressive physical therapy protocols and modified training schedules yield good results. However, the prognosis for these animals to ever reach their full genetic athletic potential is often guarded.

When detected early, the animal is rested immediately and cold therapy is initiated. After 24 hours, alternating cold and infrared therapeutic heat sessions are applied. When exercise is again an option, pre-warm the animal first before any exercise is undertaken.

Chronic cases have to be maintained with an aggressive infrared therapeutic heat program. Pre-warm the animal before exercise and repeat the infrared therapy sessions numerous times throughout the day. Those cases that are periarticular or articular are usually nonrewarding when considering treatment.

Hindlimb Disorders:

Below the stifle joint, the main source of lameness disorders within the hindlimb is the hock or tarsal joint. Distal to the hock, the soft tissues suffer some of the strains and disorders of their counterparts within the forelimb and are addressed in the same manner. However, the disorders of the hock will benefit from infrared therapeutic heat.

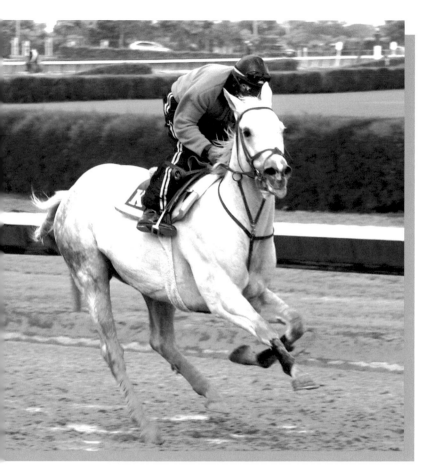

Chapter 4

Bone spavin, curbs, cunean bursitis, capped hocks, degenerative joint disease and ***osteochondrosis*** are all lameness disorders of the tarsal joint and its surrounding soft tissue. Before any treatment program is initiated, it is important to have an accurate diagnosis and a sound multimodality treatment plan in place.

Bone spavin is a condition of osteoarthritis and osteitis of the tarsal bones of the hock. This is a degenerative condition that can eventually lead to an ***ankylosis*** or fusion of the joints within the hock.

This disorder is quite common in standardbreds and the first indication that the problem exists is the animal will exercise "on the line." This means that the animal is not pacing or trotting straight in the cart but that the hindquarters are moving towards the shaft of the cart either towards or away from the affected side.

Systemic and ***intraarticular*** treatment should be coupled with an aggressive physical therapy program in these cases of bone spavin. Infrared therapeutic heat will decrease the viscosity of the joint fluid, and provide more extensibility to the tendonous and ligamentous structures within this anatomical area. The increased circulation within the tissues will also provide analgesia. A hypothetical protocol to follow at the first sign of the disorder is as follows:

- Pre-exercise warm-up for 30 minutes.
- After exercise, cold hydrotherapy to the joint and its surrounding tissues.
- Several hours later, a second treatment of infrared therapeutic heat.

Conformational challenges predispose the animal to *curbs*. A "curb" is a sprain to the tarsal plantar ligament. The clinical sign of this disorder is a visual swelling on the plantar aspect of the hock distal to the point of the hock. When palpated, there is usually heat and swelling present in these soft tissues.

The goal of the physical therapy aspect of treating this disorder is to reduce the swelling, provide analgesia and restore the tissues to a normal state. Unfortunately, once this injury occurs, it often becomes chronic and requires therapy on a daily basis.

When the first evidence of swelling occurs, apply therapeutic heat for at least 30 – 60 minutes duration. This should be done several times during a 24-hour period. Before any exercise, these tissues should receive a treatment of therapeutic heat to provide maximum flexibility for a period of at least 30 minutes. After exercise, cold hydrotherapy can be applied to the tissues followed by an infrared therapeutic heat treatment later in the day.

Cunean bursitis is an inflammatory reaction within the *cunean bursa*, cunean tendon and all of the associated soft tissue structures around the distal intertarsal and tarsometatarsal joints. The most common etiology for this disorder is improper training: "too fast, too soon." This training is often coupled with improper shoeing and a conformationally challenged horse.

An aggressive physical therapy program utilizing infrared therapeutic heat together with a reconditioning period in the training program will allow an almost complete recovery from this injury.

After an accurate diagnosis is made, the animal is rested and several infrared therapy sessions of at least 30 minutes duration are conducted daily. Often systemic and intrabursal therapy is done concurrently to speed the healing process. After the pain is gone and adequate time is given for recovery, these animals should always be warmed before any exercise session.

Chapter 4

Teaching Tip

Infrared heat therapy sessions should be at least one hour in duration when treating an athletic injury.

A *capped hock* is a visible subcutaneous swelling at the point of the hock. It is a hydroma or a traumatic bursitis that usually results from an animal kicking either in the stall or trailer.

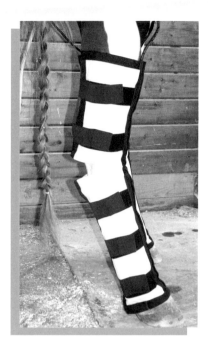

The goal of infrared therapeutic heat therapy to these cases is to reduce the swelling within the tissues. Since most of these animals are "kickers," care must be taken in introducing these animals to this modality. Once the animal realizes that this feels good, therapy sessions of 30 – 60 minutes will reduce these cosmetic blemishes.

Osteochondrosis of the tarsal bones is a failure of the developing cartilage cells to form good solid bone. These areas of inadequate bony development cannot withstand the stresses placed upon them as solid bony tissue would. This results in pain and inflammation within the joint.

Conservative treatment of these lesions includes systemic and intraarticular therapy coupled with an aggressive physical therapy program. In severe cases, arthroscopic surgery is required to help resolve this severe lameness issue.

Infrared therapeutic heat will allow the joint fluid to be more lubricative, reduce the swelling and alleviate the pain within the joint. Therapy sessions will have to be tailored on an individual case basis but should include several sessions per day. If surgery is undertaken to resolve the issue, several days after surgery infrared heat therapy can be utilized to speed the recovery.

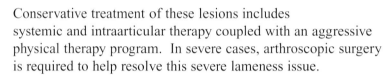

Conclusions:

Several key points are offered to summarize the numerous uses of the Thermotex™ Infrared Therapy System Leggings:

- Pre-exercise warm-up of the equine athlete is beneficial in preventing injuries, preventing re-injuries and allowing a more efficient exercise session or optimum performance in an event.
- Maintenance therapy sessions should be done on at least a daily basis.
- Treatment should only be initiated after an accurate diagnosis is made.
- Multiple sessions within a 24-hour period are beneficial.
- In an acute case, alternating cold therapy with infrared heat therapy really speeds the recovery process.

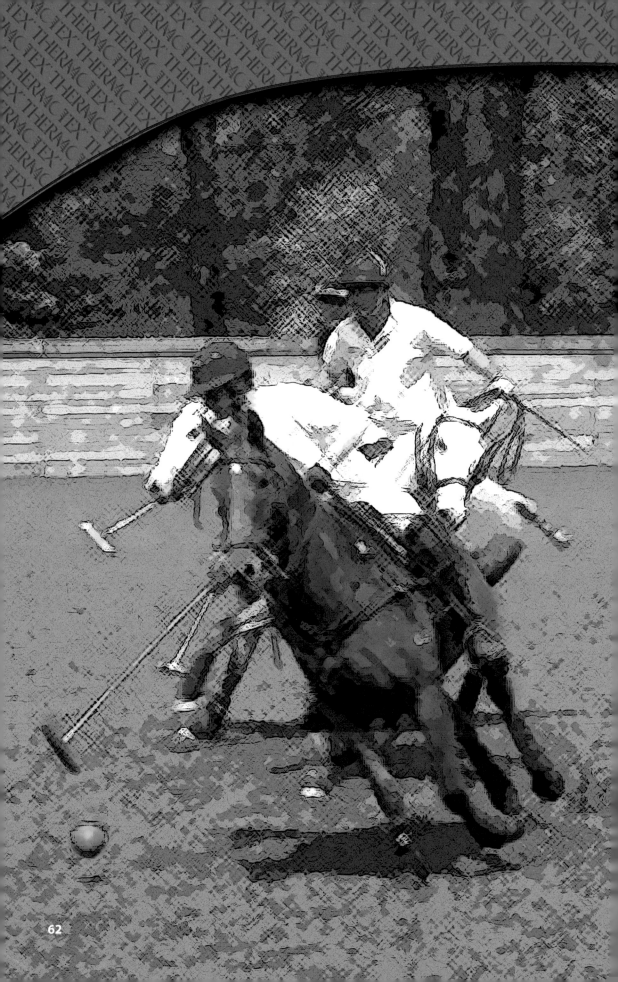

CHAPTER FIVE

Basic Therapeutic Treatment Protocols Using the Thermotex™ ITS Neck Appliance

Introduction:

The Thermotex™ Infrared Therapy System neck appliance is a two element wrap that is designed to provide three element positions on each side of the neck. It is built with the same washable tear-resistant material as the therapy blanket and is secured with three broad Velcro straps that allow application to even the largest of horses.

The three positions within the wrap for the placement of the heating elements makes this a unique infrared heating appliance. The top position allows the deep penetrating infrared heat to be applied directly over the dorsal musculature and nuchal ligament. At the base of the skull, this top position is directly over the first

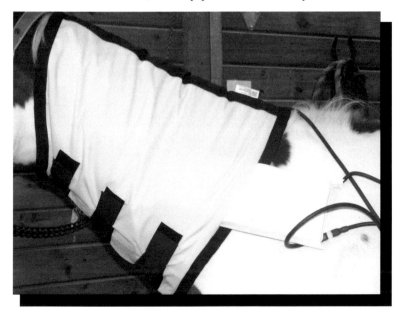

Thermotex™ ITS Neck Appliance

few cervical vertebrae. The lower positions allow the direct application of infrared therapeutic heat to the lower portions of the cervical spine and the main musculature of the neck.

The heating elements within this appliance can be applied to other anatomical areas as well. Proper positioning of the wrap allows infrared heat treatment to the upper throat area and even over the anatomical areas surrounding the jugular veins. This wrap can be attached to the therapy blanket for the application of heat to the chest area. Individually traumatized areas can easily be treated with this two-element wrap.

The physiological effects upon the horse are the same with this appliance as they are with all of the other Thermotex™ appliances. They are:

- Vasodilatation and an increase in circulation throughout all of the heated tissues.
- Pain relief.
- Increased extensibility within all of the tendons and ligaments.
- Decrease in joint stiffness.

To achieve these desired physiological effects, the neck appliance must be applied properly and often enough to achieve the desired results. The application of infrared therapeutic heat to the neck area should be long in duration – at least 30 minutes with treatment times of 45 – 60 minutes even being better. This appliance is very safe and will not burn or *dehydrate* the animal.

Equipment and Patient Basics When Using the Thermotex™ ITS Neck Appliance:

Follow these simple common sense guidelines when utilizing the neck appliance:

1. The animal should be in cross-ties and be clean.
2. All neck sweats or liniments should be removed before applying the neck appliance.
3. Pre-warm the appliance by plugging in on the high setting for a few minutes before placing on the patient.
4. Place the appliance on the neck of the animal, secure in place with the Velcro straps and position the heating elements where desired.

> ### Teaching Tip
>
> Chiropractic adjustments of cervical spinal subluxations are easily accomplished after an infrared heat therapy session of at least 45 minutes.

5. Turn the neck appliance on the high setting for the first 10 – 15 minutes of therapy. Then turn the setting to low for the remainder of the therapy session.

6. Make sure all of the electric cords are out of the reach of the animal during the entire therapy session.

6. When the therapy is concluded, wipe the inside of the wrap with a mild disinfectant, dry and store in a clean place.

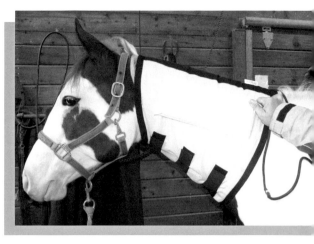

Each element has three different positions available on each side of the neck.

Using the Thermotex™ Infrared Therapy System Neck Appliance as a Pre-Event Warm-Up:

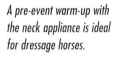

Pleasure horses, Hunters, Jumpers, Eventers, Endurance horses and especially Dressage athletes all will benefit by a pre-exercise/pre-event warm-up with the Thermotex™ Infrared Therapy System neck appliance. Ideal therapy sessions should be as follows:

A pre-event warm-up with the neck appliance is ideal for dressage horses.

- With the heating elements in the highest position: 10 – 15 minutes on the high setting and another 10 minutes on low.

- With the heating elements in the middle position: 10 minutes on the high setting and then 10 minutes on low.

- With the heating elements placed in the lowest position: 10 minutes on high and 10 minutes on low.

- After completion of this therapy session, it would be ideal to provide a massage session that would conclude with a series of neck stretches.

All equine athletes would benefit from an infrared therapy session to their neck regardless of their specific discipline.

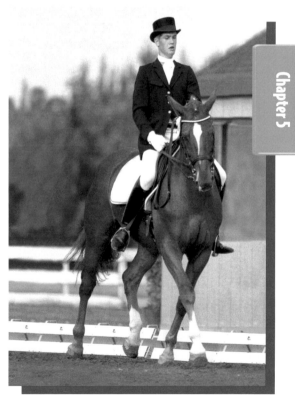

Using the Thermotex™ Infrared Therapy System Neck Appliance in a Daily Maintenance Program:

Daily infrared therapeutic heat therapy sessions prevent injuries and allow the equine athlete to perform and train comfortably and at the highest levels. The following hypothetical daily program is easy to follow and can easily be combined when using the therapeutic blanket and/or leggings:

- Quick and easy: Pre-warm the appliance and place the heating elements in the middle position of the wrap. Turn the elements onto the highest setting for 15 minutes and then low for another 15 minutes.

- Slower and more thorough: Pre-warm the appliance and place the heating elements in each of the positions, on the high setting, for a period of 15 minutes each.

- Always try to follow a therapeutic heat session with massage and stretching.

Using the Thermotex™ Infrared Therapy System Neck Appliance to Treat Various Disorders:

Localized trauma to the neck (or any other anatomical area):

Secure the neck appliance so that both of the heating elements come in direct contact with the desired area. Always pre-warm the appliance before applying. If the area is painful, i.e. localized cellulitis from an intramuscular injection, be patient and kind. Start on the low setting and only use the high setting when common sense dictates.

Abscesses:

The application of infrared therapeutic heat will bring an abscess to a head and allow the tissue to heal faster. Be patient since the application of heat to this area may be painful to the horse. Remember to clean the appliance thoroughly before storing.

Phlebitis:

Unfortunately there are occasions where an animal must receive numerous intravenous injections within the jugular vein. This results in a localized phlebitis or inflammation within the surrounding tissues of the vein. The application of infrared therapeutic heat aids in the resolution of this problem. Simply place the wrap upside down on the neck of the horse. In this way you can position the heating pads directly over the veins and their surrounding tissues. Treatment should be long and numerous times during the day when this problem exists.

Hypothermia/Shock:

After placing an I.V. catheter for the administration of fluids, a few wraps with an elastic bandage holds the catheter in place. The heat appliance can be applied over the top of this to not only secure the catheter but also provide warmth to the circulating blood within the jugular veins.

Muscle Strains of the Chest:

The neck appliance is easily applied to the chest musculature. It can be held in place using a regular stable blanket or used in combination with the Thermotex™ therapy blanket. This allows for the application of deep penetrating infrared heat to the chest musculature. Pre-warm the appliance and start the therapy session on the high setting.

Other Uses of the Thermotex™ Infrared Therapy System Neck Appliance:

There are many uses for the convenient easy-to-use neck appliance. Only our lack of imagination limits its applications. The following are just a few ideas:

Neck Sweat:

In the show ring it is desirous for the animals to have a lean looking flexible neck free of any fat deposits. Many products have been developed over the years to facilitate this goal. The Thermotex™ Infrared Therapy System neck appliance is an easy efficient way of accomplishing this goal without the risk of burning the skin, overheating or dehydration. Apply the neck wrap in the desired position and place on the low setting. Over the top of the neck appliance place a heavy neck blanket that is held in place by the halter and possibly a stable sheet. This can be left in place for hours or until the desired effect is reached.

Chiropractic adjustment:

The neck appliance allows easy manipulation of the cervical spine. A long therapy session with the hood appliance, neck appliance and therapy blanket before chiropractic therapy is performed allows for easy adjustment of the entire animal.

The neck appliance can be used as a neck sweat.

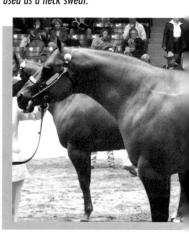

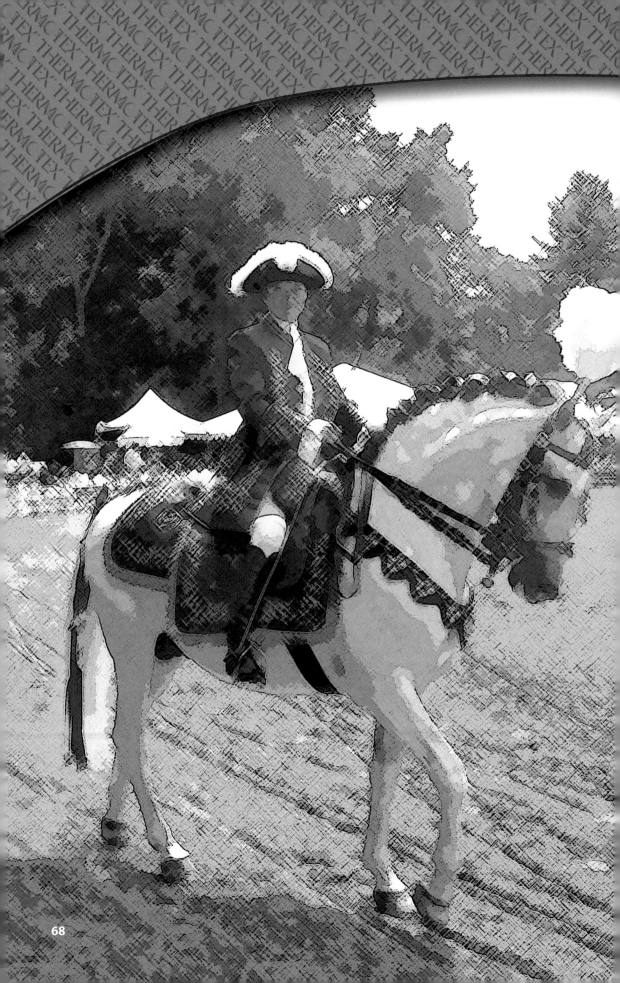

Basic Therapeutic Treatment Protocols Using the Thermotex™ ITS Hood Appliance

Introduction:

The Thermotex™ Infrared Therapy System hood appliance contains two infrared heating elements. One is located for positioning over the frontal sinuses and the other over the throat and between the lower *mandibles*. The hood is large enough to fit even the largest of breeds due to the totally adjustable portion that fits over the throat. It is made of the same durable material as the blanket and other infrared heating appliances.

A great number of equine athletes suffer from upper respiratory problems during their careers. They are highly stressed individuals and are constantly exposed to bacteria and viruses on the competitive circuit. The Thermotex™ Infrared Therapy System hood appliance provides an easy way to apply deep penetrating infrared heat to the anatomical areas of the frontal *sinuses* and throat. It is difficult to be competitive if the animal suffers from an upper respiratory disorder.

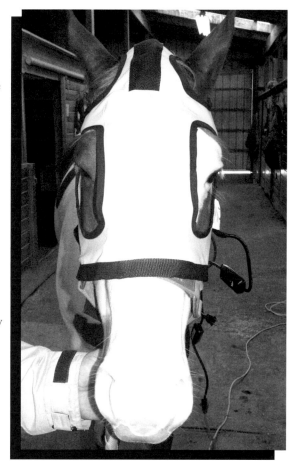

Thermotex™ ITS Hood Appliance

Chapter 6

Using the Thermotex™ ITS Hood Appliance for the Treatment of Respiratory Disorders:

Bacterial Sinusitis:

Bacterial infections of the frontal *sinuses* can be either primary in nature or secondary to an infected tooth. There is almost always pain over the frontal sinuses and the animal will have difficulty breathing. In severe cases, the animal may even show neurological signs. Radiographs and an endoscopic examination will ensure an accurate diagnosis.

Treatment plans for this disorder can be very aggressive and systematic. They may include lavage, systemic therapy, *nebulization* and even surgery. Regardless of the severity of the disorder, the application of infrared heat to the frontal sinuses has some benefit. This infrared heat will increase the circulation to the area and alleviate some of the pain and discomfort associated with this disorder. Applications, with a pre-warmed unit, should last for a minimum of 60 minutes per therapy session. These can be repeated several times a day.

> ### Teaching Tip
>
> Infrared therapy sessions with this appliance should be long in duration and applied several times a day.

Pharyngeal Lymphoid Hyperplasia: ("pimples/blisters")

The cause of these lesions is still a matter of controversy. It may be from a virus, irritants in the air, allergies or a low-grade bacterial infection. They are found on endoscopic examination and even their significance is under constant scrutiny. Some equine athletes seem to perform poorly when these structures are in evidence while still others affected similarly enter the winner's circle.

Treatment of this disorder varies from simple rest to cryosurgery. In the middle are treatments of chemical *cautery*, *electrocautery*, nebulization, systemic anti-inflammatories and antibiotics.

> ### Did you know?
>
> *Second to lameness problems, upper respiratory problems are the next leading cause for failure to achieve athletic potential.*

Chapter 6

The application of the Thermotex™ Infrared Therapy System hood appliance with the throat pad in place would certainly provide some benefit to those patients whose airflow seems to be restricted by these structures. Long therapy sessions would benefit the patient the most with the ability to increase the circulation within the tissues and supply some pain relief to this area.

Guttural Pouch Disorders:

Due to their anatomical location, the guttural pouches are always predisposed to infections. Any infection in this area will hinder the athletic ability of the horse despite their athletic discipline.

Treatment of these infections involves systemic antibiotics, lavage and even surgery. The application of infrared heat to the area of the throat will serve as an adjunct to these traditional therapies. Numerous daily sessions, of at least an hour duration, on the low setting provides an increase within the circulation to this area. This will aid in the animal's defense against the infection.

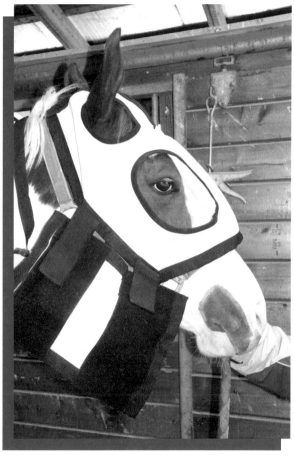

Thermotex™ ITS Hood Appliance being used to treat the Gutteral Pouch

Strangles:

This is a highly contagious infection caused by the bacteria Streptococcus equi. This bacterium usually becomes localized within the submaxillary, mandibular and retropharyngeal lymph nodes. These lymph nodes will be very painful and swell to the point where they will obstruct respiration and swallowing.

The application of infrared heat therapy to these nodes to reduce the swelling and pain is definitely of benefit to the equine patient. Therapy sessions should be conducted two to three times per day for at least 30 – 60 minutes. In most cases, the lymph nodes rupture and drain. This pustular discharge is highly contagious and care must be taken to keep it off of the Thermotex™ Infrared Therapy System hood appliance. Only use the heating element that is designed for the throat and attach it to the halter in some fashion. Wrap the entire appliance in thick disposable plastic that can be discarded after each therapy session. Even though the element is enclosed in plastic, clean after each use with a very strong disinfectant with a long contact time.

Laryngeal Hemiplegia:

The etiology of *laryngeal* hemiplegia, "roaring," is damage or irritation to the left recurrent laryngeal nerve. This causes a loss of innervation to the muscles of the larynx and a consequent loss of muscular function.

This problem is diagnosed with a thorough endoscopic exam performed after hard exercise. Surgery yields the most desirable prognosis.

The incision for this surgery is left open to heal. Daily cleaning and applications of infrared heat will speed the healing process. It is necessary to utilize the throat heating element from the hood appliance. Carefully wrap it in disposable plastic before placing it on the cleaned incision. Initially, holding the appliance on by hand is preferable to trying to tie it onto a halter

Surgical intervention for "roaring" is common in Thoroughbreds.

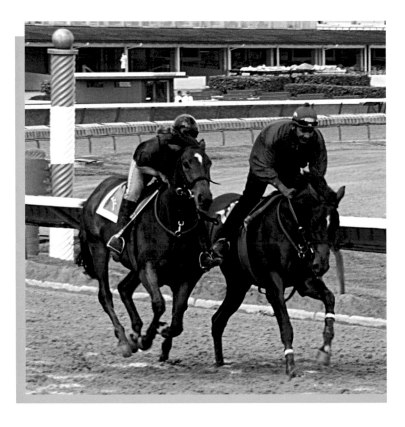

due to the tenderness of the area. After a few days, the appliance can be fixed in place for the duration of the treatment. Therapy sessions will always be on the low heat setting and for short durations immediately after surgery. As the incision heals, the length of therapy sessions will increase. Always keep the appliance clean and disinfected after each use.

Conclusions:

- The application of infrared heat to the throat area and sinuses increases the circulation and speeds the healing process.
- Infrared heat provides analgesia to the inflamed tissues within this anatomical area.
- Always protect the equipment from bacterial contamination by enclosing it in plastic and applying disinfectant after use.
- Treatment times in these areas should last at least 30-60 minutes and can be repeated several times within a 24 hour period.

Chapter 6

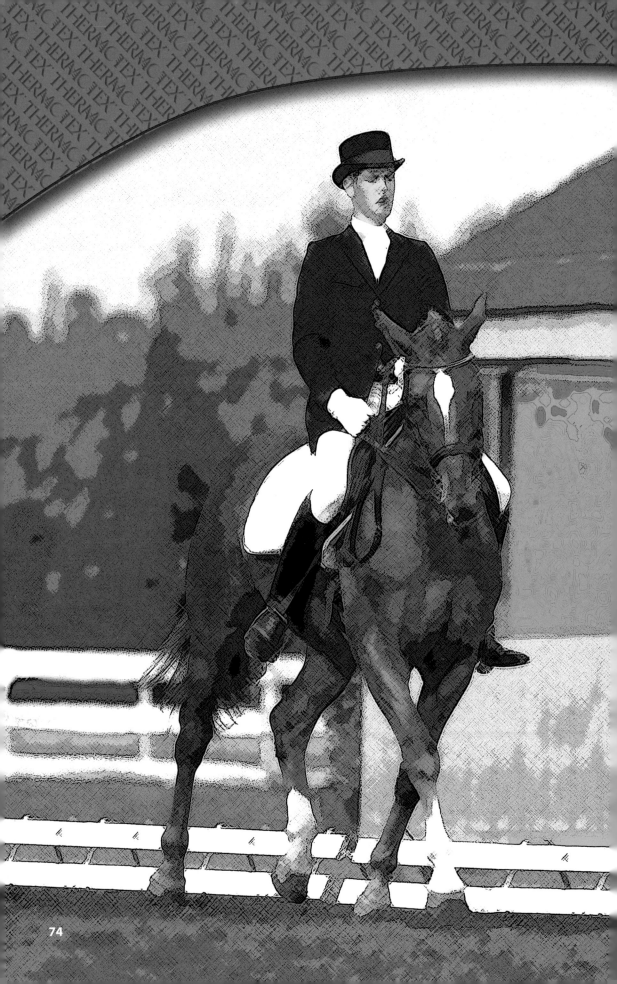

Basic Therapeutic Treatment Protocols for TMJ Using the Thermotex™ TMJ Hood

by: Todd Williams

Introduction:

The temporomandibular joint (TMJ) or jaw joint is a critical joint in the proper functional, performance and quality of life of a horse. Stress and joint pain can be demonstrated in horses. A reduction in joint function is easy for a competent horse dentist and most owners to assess. As an aid to the treatment of the temporomandibular joint dysfunction the Thermotex TMJ hood is extremely effective. The hood is designed with two heat elements that are directly over the TMJ of the horse and also has two elements over the muscles of the upper part of the neck. The intention in the placement of the primary elements is to provide penetrating heat to the affected joints and aid in the relief of stress and connective tissue pain in and around the joint. The elements on the neck of the horse aid in the relaxation and softening of the muscles of the poll of the horse. These muscles are usually affected when a horse is suffering from temporomandibular joint dysfunction.

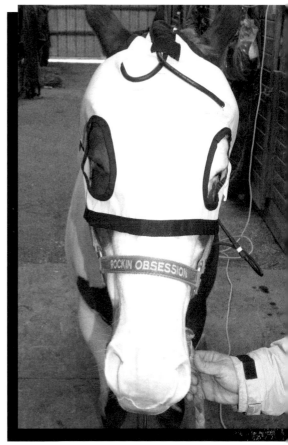

Thermotex™ ITS TMJ Hood Appliance

Temporomandibular Joint Function in the Horse:

It must first be stated that there has been minimal scientific investigation into TMJ of the horse. Much of the information available is from comparisons with human TMJ issues and a theoretical bio-mechanical model. Field work with horses, their teeth and their TM joints over the past 15 years also helps to provide clues as to TMJ function and the related issues of bits and performance. This is an area that could provide many answers to neck, back, gait, and psychological issues for the horse. All of these obviously affect the performance of the equine athlete. Horse TMJ issues are unique because we use their mouth and jaw as a communication point. The interaction of the bit and the TMJ is crucial to high-level function of the horse in any competition. If the TMJ is dysfunctional or painful and the bit is moved to the left or right then the jaw receives lateral pressure to move in that direction. This movement requires the left and right jaw joints to move in very different ways. Pain reaction in the TMJ may be responsible for the horse resisting the directional cue. The hesitation involved can make the difference to a first place finish and some other less desirable outcome. The term "collection" is found frequently in the horse industry and is used to describe a very specific posture in the horse. Proper posture and the relationship of the TMJ are uniquely tied in both humans and horses. Substantial evidence and understanding of this posture indicates that it is primary to many of the movements that are actively sought by most

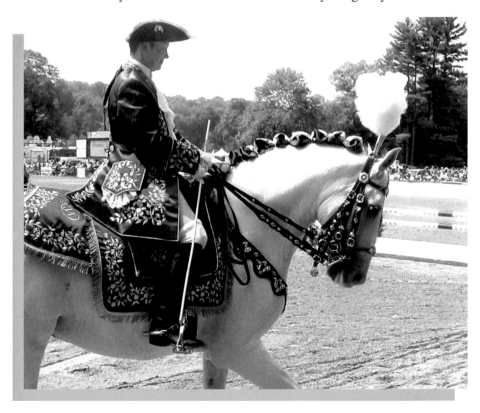

Basic Therapeutic Treatment Protocols for TMJ

competitors in the equine world. The ease with which a horse can be collected may rely heavily on correct TMJ function.

Typical Case Study A middle aged Saddle horse was presented for treatment. The initial evaluation was difficult and the mare exhibited a serious pain response when the jaw joints were palpated as well as a moderately high level of dental pathology. The mare was flighty and difficult to deal with initially and could only be managed with the aid of sedative drugs. A full dental workup to correct the mare's mouth pathology was undertaken. The treatment included the reduction of dominant cheek teeth and proper shaping and balancing

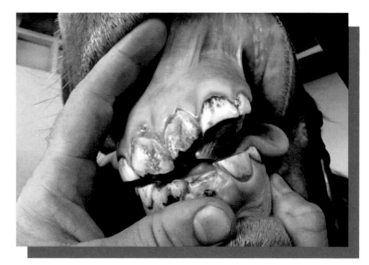

of the grinding teeth (premolars and molars). A full incisor equilibration was required to establish correct mouth function. The mare's mouth was brought up to 100% of its functional potential. The aim of this treatment plan was to eliminate any conflict between the three main parts of the dental apparatus. Part 1 is the jaw joint, part 2 is the muscles of mastication and part 3 is the teeth. At the conclusion of the treatment the Thermotex TMJ hood was used on the mare to facilitate her recovery from the changes in her mouth and reduce any pain in the joints. One of the complaints of the owner was the inability to keep the mare on a 12-meter circle. This was critical to the performance demands that were being placed on the horse.

Within a week there was a considerable change in the function of the jaw and the temperament and performance levels of the mare. The mare was more calm and able to work comfortably with proper posture and maintain the circle. More significantly the attitude change and flighty behavior was very noticeably reduced. Much of the improvement in performance and attitude is likely derived from the improved joint function. The mare would have benefited from the direct reduction of pain in the mouth but this specific treatment centered on providing proper mouth balance and function. Proper "three-point" balance and function is based on the TMJ as one of the three specific points.

> **Teaching Tip**
>
> A thorough dental exam should be included in all lameness examinations.

Chapter 7

Temporomandibular Joint Anatomy & Function:

The jaw or mandible of the horse is one continuous piece of bone with a pair of hinges or joints at either end. These joints act independently, that is, they seldom make identical movements during normal mastication, or performance. The

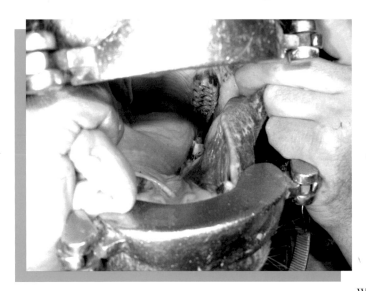

A dental exam aided by the use of a speculum.

simple movement of the jaw of the horse laterally requires one joint to pivot on an axis vertically through the joint while the opposite joint may have to translate forward to facilitate this movement. What is crucial is that the joints are symmetrical in their form as well as their function. If the joints allow the jaw to swing 25 mm to the horses left (near side) then there must also be a swing of 25 mm to the right (off side) of the horse. This will help keep the movement and performance of the horse balanced and the dental pathology to a minimum. This can be facilitated by the use of deep penetrating but low temperature heat on these joints. This is exactly what the Thermotex products provide.

The mouth of the horse is designed with teeth that develop long extended crowns that are stored in the horse's head. This is called the reserve crown because it is held in reserve and extrudes, as there is attrition to the part of the tooth that is in use in the mouth. The tooth that is in use in the oral cavity is called the clinical crown and is generally the part that we work on in clinic. Both the incisors and the grinding teeth or cheek teeth continuously extrude. This creates the potential for an imbalance to be created if the two parts do not wear evenly. The imbalance may be responsible for pressure changes in the TMJ. Proper occlusion or contact of the grinders or cheek teeth is the issue that is in question. Horses are designed to have contact on their back grinding teeth just as humans are designed to have contact on their grinding teeth. If an imbalance occurs then there is reason to expect that the horse will experience discomfort in the jaw joints. This is evidenced in clinical examinations.

Equine Dentistry:

It would be difficult to discuss the treatment of the TMJ without discussion of the treatment of teeth in the horse. As with human dentistry dental treatments in the horse can result in conflicts between the muscles, joint and teeth. The first rule of dentistry regardless of the species being worked on is to resolve this conflict. In the past 5 years there has been an increase in the use of power tools to float teeth. This method usually involves devices to hang the head of the horse for the benefit of the dental practitioner. These changes in treatment methods have resulted in a large-scale

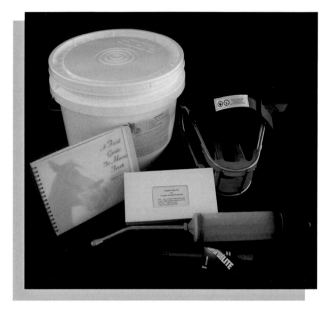

Crystal Animal Products

problem that did not exist when everyone used only handheld files to perform dental work. Many horses hung in cradles or as one supplier calls them "cranial support stands" while sedated show marked pain and reactivity in the TMJ and neck after this method of treatment. The repair of horses that were injured by the head hanging/headstand techniques is one of the factors that brought us to the design of the Thermotex TMJ hood. The hood has now proven its worth as an aid to the repair and therapy for this group of horses. It is also useful after any reconstructive dentistry where the horse is likely to feel discomfort from occlusal adjustments and changes to the mouth of the horse. If a headstand is to be used in performing horse dentistry then I strongly recommend that the hood be used as a means of reducing the pain in the joints that will result.

Because of the critical nature of this joint, providing therapy for it would be beneficial to most performance horses. To optimize the success of the Thermotex based TMJ therapy, the hood should be used as an addition to competent dentistry for the horse. The ideology behind the dental work must be function based and applied consistently and individually to each horse. For more information on dentistry and to learn how to evaluate your horse's mouth, a kit is available from Crystal Animal Products. *(www.crystalanimalproducts.com)*

Therapeutic Effects:

The effect of the heat applied with a TMJ hood is to reduce inflammation in the connective tissues surrounding the joint. This is the main compelling feature of the treatment protocol. Reduction of pain will help the horse to increase the lateral movement of the jaw, in other words increasing the range of motion of the joint. This increased range of movement then improves the overall function to the joint and its connective tissue as well as the general function of the masticatory machinery of the horse. As the horse is better able to relax in its jaw and neck a direct translation into improved performance is obvious. Better head sets and easier flexion at the poll will improve the gait and stance of the horse. The therapeutic effect of the TMJ hood is again enhanced by competent dental work that goes beyond regular rasping of sharp points and is designed to promote proper mouth function.

Basic Treatment Protocols:

The basic treatment protocol is to pre-heat the Thermotex hood on high, to bring it up to temperature. The horse should be clean and dried on the area that is to be treated and free from dirt. The horse should be monitored during this time, as it is possible for the animal to become uncomfortable with the hood on. After initial warm up place the hood on the head of the horse insuring that the electric cords will not become entangled or stepped on. In most cases 20 minutes of therapy on the joints is sufficient to provide the level of analgesia to facilitate the normal use of the joint. These treatments may be repeated as frequently as required by the horse to relieve pain. In most cases 7 to 10 treatments seem to be sufficient. Feeding the horse a mash when the hood is removed helps to get the joints moving. Alternately a massage and gentle manipulation of the jaw will aid in increasing the mobility of joints. A second use for the performance horse is as a warm up for the joint prior to a work out or training session. Current evidence suggests that warming the TMJ prior to work will noticeably improve performance. This is an ongoing treatment or therapy and can be done as a daily routine.

The Thermotex TMJ hood is easy to use and provides a very effective way to provide therapy to a difficult area of the horse.

.Conclusions:

- A pain free TMJ is critical in maintaining the athletic potential in the equine athlete.

- A pain free TMJ allows for easier collection.

- The Thermotex™ Infrared Therapy System TMJ hood provides analgesia to the TMJ and reduces the inflammation within the surrounding connective tissues.

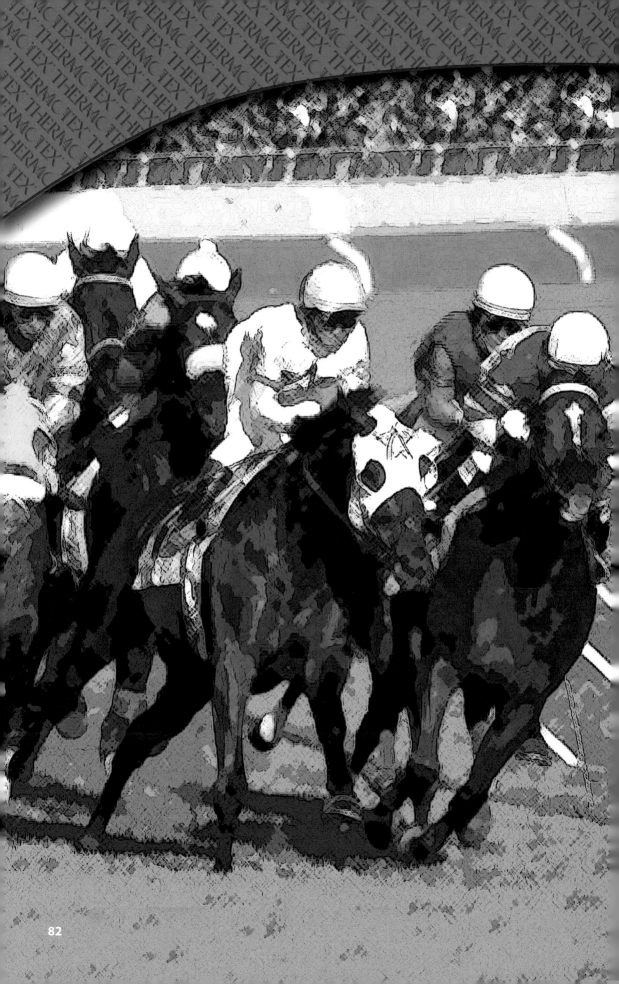

Basic Therapeutic Treatment Protocols Using the Thermotex™ ITS Appliances for each Discipline

Introduction:

Breed characteristics and conformation determine the physical ability a particular horse has to perform within a specific discipline. Thoroughbreds excel in dressage, hunting, jumping, eventing and racing whereas Arabians excel in showing under saddle and endurance. Warmbloods are quite capable of performing dressage, hunting, jumping and eventing whereas Appaloosas and Paints do extremely well in western performance and endurance.

Each discipline requires the best of the horse's ability to compete at a high level within that discipline. The horse must use its entire musculoskeletal system in performing its specific

Standardbred racing below. Opposite page: flat racing.

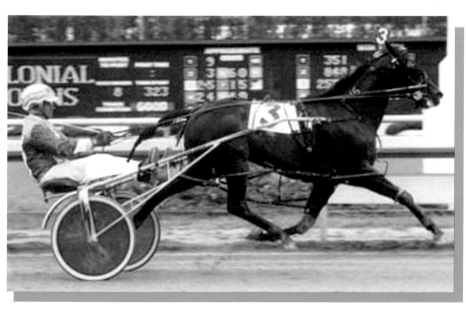

discipline. Yet, each discipline places its own unique stresses upon the horse specific to its event. Use of the Thermotex™ Infrared Therapy System appliances will allow a horse to compete when relaxed, flexible and at the peak of its individual performance capability.

Protocols for each discipline vary when using the Thermotex™ Infrared Therapy System appliances. The goal is to focus on the anatomical areas of stress characteristic of that discipline to maximize the performance. However, if a clinical problem exists, consult a veterinarian before treatment is initiated.

Arabians excel in showing under saddle and endurance riding.

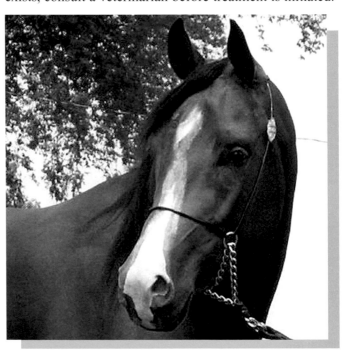

Teaching Tip

Each discipline places stress upon different anatomical areas. Each of these areas would benefit from the application of infrared heat.

General Guidelines:

The therapeutic effects of infrared heat to the various anatomical areas of the horse are the same as mentioned throughout this text. They are:

- Vasodilatation and increased blood flow throughout all of the tissues.

- Analgesia.

- Increased extensibility within the ligaments and tendons.

- Decrease in joint stiffness.

- The psychological effect on the horse by allowing relaxation and a relief from stress.

The following general step-by-step guidelines should be considered when applying this unique modality to any area of the horse:

1. The horse should have its head tied up or be placed in a set of cross-ties. In some cases a muzzle will need to be utilized. This ensures safety from the electrical requirement of the appliances.

2. All dirt, poultice, liniments or any topically applied substances should be removed from the limbs or any other anatomical area either by brushing or with a hose and water.

3. Pre-warm the appliance before placing it on the animal.

4. Turn the switch to the low setting initially until the animal becomes acquainted with the therapy. After a few minutes, set the switch on high for at least 10 - 15 minutes.

5. Continue the therapy at the low setting for the duration of the treatment.

6. When the treatment is concluded, the inside of the appliance should be wiped down with a mild disinfectant, dried and stored in a clean place.

Guidelines for Using Thermotex™ Appliances For Each Specific Discipline:

The daily rigors of show jumping competition can take their toll on the athletes.

JUMPERS

Show or stadium jumping requires a horse to jump over a challenging course usually in the shortest time possible with the fewest faults. A single rail or a few tenths of a second often determine the final standings within this discipline. The animals that compete successfully in this event require agility, balance, control and an incredible amount of power from the musculoskeletal system.

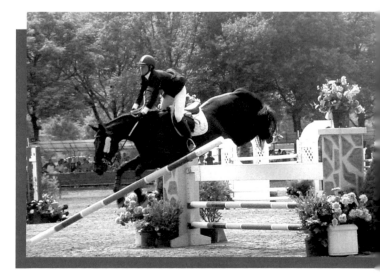

The application of infrared therapeutic heat is beneficial as a part of the pre-event warm-up, maintenance of peak performance and as a treatment upon a clinical disorder. Each unique situation has to be evaluated upon its own merits and addressed on an individual basis.

There are several areas of stress within these athletes that would benefit from infrared therapeutic heat. The take-off or initiation of the jump places a great deal of strain upon flexors, extensor muscles, tendons and ligaments of the hindquarters. The landing places a great deal of strain upon the flexor muscles, tendons and ligaments of the forelimb, the shoulder, chest and back. The impact even causes a tension within the neck.

Pre-event warm-up of the jumper:

- Application of the therapy blanket for at least 30 – 45 minutes before exercise or other pre-event procedures.
- Application of the neck appliance for 30 minutes before the event.
- Application of a set of leggings to both the front and hind legs for 30 minutes before exercise.
- Following the application of infrared heat, massage or any other modality can be utilized to further prepare this equine athlete for competition.

General maintenance of the jumper:

- Application of the therapy blanket for at least 30 – 60 minutes on a daily basis before exercise.

- Application of the therapy blanket for a second treatment in the late afternoon or evening after a particularly hard training session.

- Application of the leggings for at least 30 minutes to both the front and hind limbs on a daily basis.

Treatment of the jumper:

- Before any treatment regime is initiated, an accurate diagnosis of the problem is essential.

- Generalized muscle soreness responds well to several lengthy treatments in a 24-hour period. These therapy sessions should last a minimum of 30 minutes each and can continue for as long as an hour in duration.

- Most tendon and ligament injuries respond well to a therapy program consisting of alternating heat and cold treatments. This speeds the

The take-off phase of the jump places incredible strain on the structures of the hindquarters.

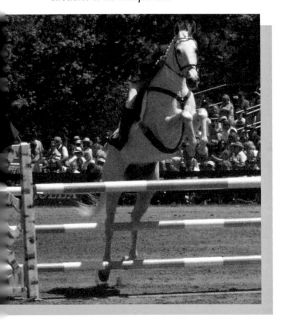

healing processes tremendously. After cold therapy is applied, wait a period of time before initiating heat treatments. Infrared heat treatments can last up to an hour in duration, several times within a 24-hour period.

- The versatility of the Thermotex™ Infrared Therapy System appliances allows the use of even a single pad upon a specific anatomical area for treatment. A single pad can be placed upon an area such as the chest and held in place by using Velcro or bandages using the infrared therapy blanket as the supporting structure.

HUNTERS

To successfully compete in this event, these equine athletes need to be agile, sound, have good manners around hounds and other horses and exhibit a great deal of strength and stamina. Those horses used in field hunting and fox hunting are usually Thoroughbreds, Irish drafts or Warmbloods.

In the show ring, the hunter classes are not as strenuous but still require strength and agility under control. Horses chosen for this discipline are usually Quarter Horses, Thoroughbreds, Warmbloods or crosses of these three.

Hunters can compete in the show ring or in the field on a wide variety of surfaces and terrain.

Field hunters compete upon an uneven and mostly rough terrain. This puts a stress upon the legs of the animal. When these animals are asked to jump obstacles along the course, they place the same type of stresses upon their anatomy that a show jumper would except they often land on a variety of uneven surfaces. In the show ring, the type of class the animal competes in will determine the types of stress placed on the animal.

Pre-event warm-up, daily maintenance and treatment of the Hunter: The programs outlined for the jumpers are easily applied to the Hunter. The pre-event warm-up cannot be too long in nature and should last at least one hour. This event is different from the

Did you know?

Equine Athletes perform to the best of their abilities following thorough pre-event warm-up protocols.

show or stadium jumping since the animals land on an uneven surface. The more flexible and agile the animal is, the less likely an injury will occur. Maintenance therapy is focused upon relief of any areas of primary soreness or secondary soreness from stresses caused by problems within the limbs. Treatments should follow an accurate diagnosis and be aimed at not only the primary source of lameness but also any secondary sources arising from a primary source. An example of this is a stone bruise causing a stress upon the musculature of the shoulder. The stone bruise is addressed in its own capacity and the shoulder soreness would benefit from application of the Thermotex™ Infrared Therapy System blanket for several treatments.

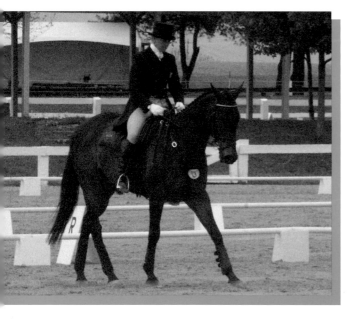

Upper level dressage horses place high levels of stress upon their entire anatomical structure.

DRESSAGE

When one watches dressage, it is like watching poetry in motion. The horses are elegant, flexible, agile and have a certain flair and finesse in the execution of their discipline. These animals must have excellent conformation to compete at a high level and have a muscle development and carriage quite different from the high-level jumpers, hunters and eventers.

Powerful horses such as the Dutch, Danish, German and Swedish Warmbloods comprise the majority of the breeds within this discipline. However, American Warmbloods, Andalusians, Fresians, Thoroughbreds and Quarter Horses perform extremely well at dressage.

Athletic training of these animals places a high level of stress upon their entire anatomy. The back, hips, stifles and hocks have to be free moving and flexible to provide the drive needed for these events. Lateral work such as side passes and bending places a stress upon the chest. Shoulders have to be flexible and move freely. Any soreness or injury to legs that restricts extension is completely unacceptable within this discipline. Collection of the head for a proper set places stress on the muscles within the jaw area and neck until they are capable of handling the training.

Pre-event warm-up of the Dressage horse:

- Application of the Thermotex™ Infrared Therapy System therapy blanket, neck appliance and hood approximately three to four hours before the event for a period of at least 60 minutes. Each therapy program is unique to each horse as its warm-up and ability are an individual characteristic.

- The Thermotex™ Infrared Therapy System Leggings should be applied to both the hind limbs and forelimbs for a period of not less than 30 minutes each.

- After the animal is warm and supple, stretching and massage work are a great complementary therapy for these animals.

Maintenance Protocols for the Dressage Athlete: These animals need to be maintained at the highest level of fitness and be as comfortable as possible to compete in these events. The following daily guidelines will achieve this goal.

> ### Did you know?
>
> *The flexibility and agility that is required by the dressage athlete is greatly enhanced through the application of infrared heat.*

- The animal should receive infrared heat therapy over its entire anatomy for at least 45 minutes before any exercise is initiated. After this therapy is completed, it is essential that the animal be stretched through all the normal range of motion stretches. Massage techniques are applied to any specific areas of stress or soreness.

- After the animal is exercised, cooled out and allowed to relax, a second therapy is initiated with just the blanket to relieve any body soreness that may have occurred from the exercise session.

Treatment Protocols for the Dressage Athlete: Treatment of any specific disorder should not be initiated until an accurate diagnosis is made. Treatment of muscle soreness is easily accomplished by increasing the treatment time and the number of treatment sessions within a 24-hour period. Specific treatment of a lameness disorder should only be accomplished with the guidance of the attending veterinarian or an accomplished equine physical therapist.

EVENTING

Three different disciplines, each with different athletic requirements, are performed over a three day period of time. These three days consist of: dressage, cross-country and stadium jumping. Therefore, these horses undergo grueling training in all three disciplines at the same time. They are required to exhibit power, endurance, courage, intelligence, agility and strength. Both the horse and rider must have a high level of fitness and competence to compete successfully within this discipline. The breeds one is likely to find in this sport are mostly Thoroughbreds, Warmbloods, such as Hanoverians and Trakehners, and crosses.

During the strenuous training of these equine athletes there isn't a single anatomical area that would not benefit from the use of infrared therapeutic heat. All of the muscle groups, tendons, ligaments and joints experience a great deal of stress that results in inflammation and soreness.

Pre-event Warm-up of the Eventer: Each animal competing at this level will have its own unique preparation schedule. Several modalities and techniques will be used to ensure that these athletes perform at the highest level they are capable of. The general guidelines are as follows:

Did you know?

Infrared heat applied after a rigorous day of jumping can aid in the recovery of the equine athlete.

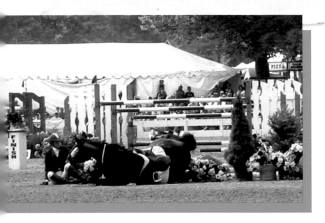

• The animal should receive a therapy session several hours before competition that should include at least 45 to 60 minutes in the therapy blanket, 30 to 45 minutes in the hood and neck appliance and 45 to 60 minutes using the leggings on both the hind and forelimbs. After this therapy session, other modalities such as massage and complete range of motion stretching should be used to prepare these athletes.

• After the first day of competition, the animal is cooled out and allowed to relax. In the evening, before the next day's event, another therapy session is beneficial to relieve any soreness and inflammation incurred on the first day.

• Several hours before the commencement of the second day's event, another therapy session is conducted in the same fashion as the first. This is tailored to fit any unique requirements that the individual athlete may have.

• After the second day of competition, the animal is rested and made comfortable. Six to eight hours later, another therapy session is initiated to prepare for the third day's event. This would generally last an hour but can be increased as needed.

- Before the third day of competition, another therapy session, with all of the appliances, will allow these animals to perform at the peak of their ability.
- After the last day, it is important to treat the animal again to allow a faster recovery from the stress incurred from the last few days of competition.

Maintenance of the Eventer:
Each one of these animals is so unique that it is difficult to generalize a routine maintenance program. Daily applications of all of the Thermotex™ Infrared Therapy System appliances would be ideal before and after a training session. Often these animals are shipped great distances and compete again after only a brief rest. These situations require a more aggressive maintenance treatment protocol than those with long periods of rest between competitions. Remember, there is a large safety margin with the Thermotex™ Infrared Therapy System appliances so overheating and dehydration are not a concern. Therefore, the more applications of the equipment, the better the therapy especially when it is combined with other modalities such as massage.

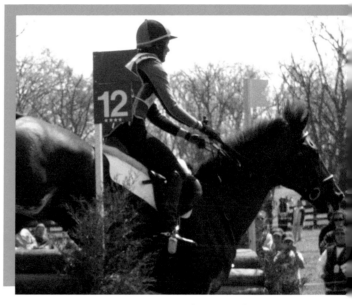

Event horses are subjected to such a great deal of stress and such unique circumstances that each individual horse should be evaluated before developing a maintenance program or treating an injury.

Treatment Protocols Involving the Eventer: These animals are subjected to so much stress and training that treatment of an injury with the Thermotex™ Infrared Therapy System appliances should only be conducted under the supervision of a veterinarian or equine physical therapist who has a unique relationship with this particular animal. In all cases an accurate diagnosis should be obtained before any treatment program is started.

Did you know?

The application of infrared heat and massage is helpful in maintaining the equine athlete between competitions.

ENDURANCE

Competitive trail riding and long distance endurance racing both fall into this category. These equine athletes are asked to cover distances of 25 to 100 miles over terrain that often includes steep hills and trails with numerous obstacles. This requires a great deal of strength and stamina from both the horse and the rider.

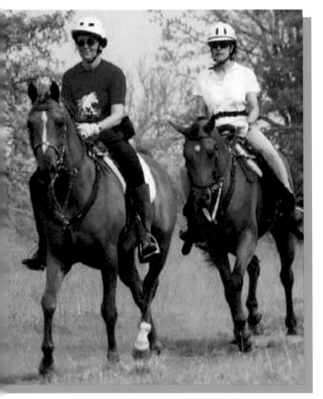

Endurance horses often cover distances up to 100 miles. This requires great stamina from both horse and rider.

Although all breeds of horses compete in endurance races, the Arabian Horse and its crosses possess the natural ability to be the most competitive.

Often these events are conducted far from electricity that makes using the Thermotex™ Infrared Therapy System appliances very difficult before these competitions. In addition, many rules apply within different associations that prohibit the use of any outside aid to the animals before a race and during the competition. The main use of the Thermotex™ Infrared Therapy System appliances within this discipline is in the recovery stage after the race and maintenance of the horses during the training period.

Recovery Protocols after an Endurance Competition: The goals of recovery therapy performed on an endurance horse are:

• An increase in the circulation within the musculature to aid in the removal of lactic acid and the byproducts of severe work upon the musculature.

• To provide comfort and pain relief.

• A relief of inflammation within the tissues and joints.

The Thermotex™ Infrared Therapy System appliances provide an easy complete modality for accomplishing these goals.

After the animal is rested, hydrated and relaxed, the Thermotex™ Infrared Therapy System therapy blanket should be applied on the low setting for 30 – 60 minutes. In addition, the leggings, neck and hood appliances can be applied as needed. These therapy sessions can be applied as often as deemed necessary for the animal to recover.

Maintenance Protocols for the Endurance Athlete: Several hours before a training session begins, a therapy session should be initiated using the therapy blanket, leggings and neck appliances. The duration of the therapy should be at least 30 minutes to allow the athlete to be well warmed–up, flexible and agile before the training even begins. This will also offer a relief of soreness from prior training sessions.

After the animal has trained, cooled out and relaxed, a second session in the evening is beneficial in the aid in recovery from the training. This is especially true where the course includes many steep hills or sand footing.

You can't overuse these therapy devices within this discipline. The more therapy sessions that are conducted, the more comfortable and happy your horse will be.

THOROUGHBRED RACEHORSES

Racing on a flat surface requires exceptional speed and stamina. Although the distances vary and the footing is of different types, the Thoroughbred breed dominates this discipline.

Comformationally, these animals are large with very long legs and long bodies. The race starts with a quick dash to establish position and then becomes an intense battle to cross the finish line. These factors predispose these animals to a great deal of stress upon the long muscles of the back, the musculature of the

Teaching Tip

Thermotex™ appliances can be used on endurance horses without fear of further dehydration.

Flat racing requires the speed and stamina for which Thoroughbreds are famous.

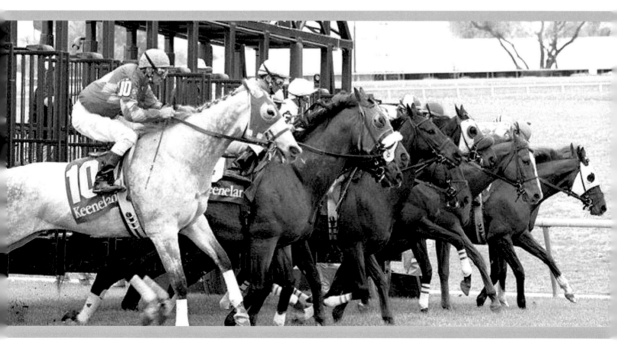

hindquarters, the neck, chest and all of the tendons and ligaments within the limbs. In addition, this intense workout leads to a lactic acid buildup within the musculature that leads to other problems within these heavily used muscles.

The goals of therapy with the Thermotex™ Infrared Therapy System appliances differ very little from other disciplines. They are:

- Increase the circulation to provide more nutrients to the muscle tissues and remove wastes such as lactic acid.
- Provide an increased flexibility so that these muscles can work with more efficiency and stamina.
- Alleviate soreness within the muscle tissue and stiffness within the joints to allow the animal to perform at its peak.

Pre-race Protocol for the Thoroughbred racehorse: As close to post time as possible, provide a therapy session with the Thermotex™ Infrared Therapy System therapy blanket, neck appliance and leggings. This should last at least 30 minutes but can last up to one hour in duration. This allows the animal to already be warmed-up before it even hits the track. Some animals exhibit nervousness the day of the race and a therapy session often has a relaxing effect upon the animal so that it can run a smart race.

Thoroughbreds are known to exhibit more nervousness on event days than other breeds. The therapy session can have a relaxing effect on the horse and improve performance.

Maintenance Protocols for the Thoroughbred racehorse: The Thermotex™ Infrared Therapy System appliances can be used in two ways to maintain a sound comfortable animal in training. Each day, the appliances can be used to warm up the athlete before any exercise begins. This allows a more flexible agile athlete that will get the most out of a training session. After a particularly hard workout or a day of long slow distance, the therapy appliances can be used to help the animal recover. This quicker recovery time maximizes the training time and allows a more efficient training program. Therapy sessions should never be less than 30 minutes and can be longer as the situation dictates.

HARNESS RACING

The Standardbred breed is the foundation of harness racing. These animals are bred for speed, endurance and stamina. These animals are either trotters or pacers. The trot is exemplified by the opposite front and rear feet propelling and landing at the same time whereas, in the pace, the front and hind feet on the same side propel and land simultaneously.

Characteristically, these animals develop soreness in the hindquarters, along the musculature of the back, throughout the shoulders, neck and at the base of the skull. These animals place stress throughout their bodies due to the harness that they wear and the repetitive gait they are required to perform each day. These animals train hard, over many miles, and often race on a weekly basis. Foundation miles, before time is a factor, often number in the 1000's.

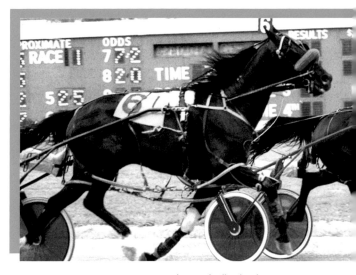

The Standardbred is the foundation of harness racing.

It is also not unusual to train an animal two trips at speed on a Tuesday, jog Wednesday, Thursday and Friday and then race on Saturday. They will have Sunday off and jog again on Monday before the entire process is repeated.

Using the hypothetical training program outlined above, the following therapy sessions would allow a more efficient training time, a sounder and more comfortable athlete and ultimately an animal that would have an edge over others in the same race:

Monday: A therapy session of at least 30 minutes in duration before the animal is taken out to jog. This can be with any of the applicable Thermotex™ Infrared Therapy System appliances but at least with the therapy blanket.

Tuesday: A therapy session of at least 30 to 60 minutes with any of the applicable Thermotex™ Infrared Therapy System appliances before the animal is taken out to train. After training, when the animal is cooled down (evening), another therapy session is initiated for at least 30 – 45 minutes to aid in the recovery.

> **Did you know?**
>
> *Minimal application of infrared heat to the Standardbred would include therapy sessions after training plus the day before and day of the race.*

Wednesday: Training would call for a light jog at slow speed. The athlete is given a therapy session that lasts approximately 30 minutes before exercise.

Thursday: A pre-exercise session is given to the animal right before jogging. A second session may be beneficial in the evening if the animal is exhibiting soreness throughout the musculature.

Friday: Light training with some speed work. Again a pre-exercise therapy session is utilized before exercise with a second session later in the day if needed.

Saturday: Race day. Before taking the animal out on the track to warm up, a therapy session is given for at least 30 minutes. The animal is then taken out to warm up for the race a little while before the actual start. Upon return to the paddock, the animal is placed in the therapy blanket and kept warm at the low setting before final preparations are made for its race.

Sunday: A therapy session may be offered to allow the animal a faster recovery from the previous day's racing.

Throughout the training program, these general principles can be applied even before the animal is training anywhere close to racing speed. Therapy sessions given on a daily basis allow a faster recovery from the rigors of training and ultimately lead to a more efficient athlete.

The "over check" portion of the harness can stress the head and neck musculature.

Because of the "over check" portion of the harness, stress is placed on the head and neck musculature. This can be adjusted if a problem exists but often is a constant area of concern and often an overlooked area for the trainer. Therapy sessions using the Thermotex™ Infrared Therapy System neck and hood appliances provide a relief of stress to these areas. Therapy sessions should last at least 30 minutes with the first 10 minutes on the high temperature setting and the remainder of the time on the low setting.

Basic Therapeutic Treatment Protocols for each Discipline

POLO

Polo ponies must be able to start fast, make abrupt turns on a dime, flying lead changes, slide to a stop and neck rein. Often times the rider is in an out-of-balance position and the animal must also compensate for this. These animals are usually less than or about 15 hands high, extremely well balanced, agile, fast, have great stamina and are very obedient.

These athletes come complete with their own unique set of stresses upon their musculoskeletal systems. They are predisposed to:

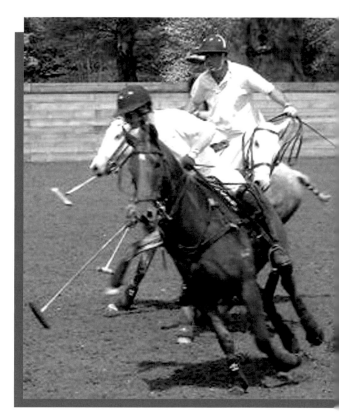

- Constant tendon strains.
- Strain upon the musculature and joints of the hindquarters.
- Strains upon the lumbosacral joint and the surrounding musculature.
- Stress upon the musculature of the neck due to the constant quick changes in direction.
- Strains upon the chest and shoulders from the abrupt stops.
- Tying up due to the lactic acid buildup within the musculature during this strenuous activity.

Pre-event warm-up of Polo Ponies: Use of the Thermotex™ Infrared Therapy System leggings (on both fore- and hindlimbs), therapy blanket sessions and treatment with the neck appliance allow for a more agile, comfortable athlete less predisposed to injury. The Polo athlete should be warmed up with at least a 30 – 60 minute therapy session before the match. This therapy session can easily become an adjunct to other modalities such as massage.

Polo ponies must compensate for the "out-of-balance" position of their riders.

Event recovery and maintenance: Therapy sessions should be performed after the animal competes and is allowed to cool down. This will aid in the recovery and allow the athlete to be more comfortable. Often it would be of benefit to use cool water on the limbs first while the therapy blanket is on the horse.

Daily maintenance will help insure a sound willing athlete during training. Sessions can be both before and after exercise for at least 30 minutes in duration.

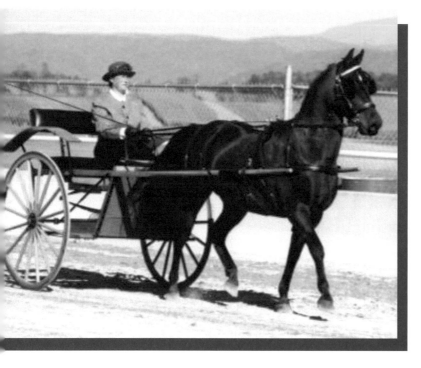
Treatment of the Polo Ponies: Treatment of the limbs of a Polo pony should never be initiated before an accurate diagnosis is made. The strain and stress to the ligaments and tendons is harsh and a treatment program should be followed in accordance with a veterinarian or equine therapist's advice. Often it is beneficial to combine a sequence of hot and cold therapies to the limbs to allow a quicker recovery.

GAITED HORSES

These athletes can be shown under saddle or in harness. Even at the rack, these animals are smooth riding and quite animated. Breeds in this category include: Tennessee Walkers, the American Saddlebred, the Missouri Fox Trotters, Paso Finos and Peruvian Pasos.

Gaited horses are shown under saddle or in harness.

Due to their animated gait, stress is applied to the musculature of the neck, shoulder and forelimb. The higher the rise of the forelimb, the better and this places its own unique stress upon the tendons and ligaments within the limb.

When these athletes are shown under saddle, the stress of the weight of the rider and the consequent change in the center of gravity and balance of the horse places stress upon the back and loin of the horse.

Daily Maintenance of the Gaited Horses: These athletes benefit from daily therapy sessions with the Thermotex™ Infrared Therapy System appliances. Therapy sessions with the hood, neck appliance, blanket and leggings provide an athlete that is much more agile and flexible in performance. Before each exercise session or class at a show, the animal should receive 30 – 60 minutes of therapy.

WESTERN PERFORMANCE ATHLETES

Western Performance events include a wide range of athletic endeavors. These events include:

- The speed and agility of the barrel racer.
- The acceleration and quick stops of the calf roper.
- The flying lead changes and slides of the reiner.
- The constant starts and stops of the cutting.
- The elegance and gait of the western pleasure classes.

Each discipline within this category has its own unique set of stresses upon the athlete and the rider. These animals all must exhibit agility, stamina, sudden bursts of speed and great reflexes. The breeds that excel at these events include Quarter Horses, Paints and Appaloosas.

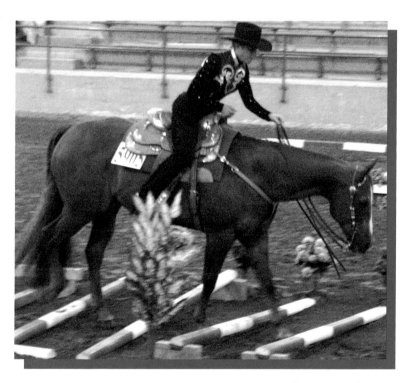

Western riding covers a wide range of disciplines accompanied by a variety of stresses for both the horse and rider.

All of these events put a great deal of stress upon the entire western performance athlete. The Reiner puts a tremendous amount of stress upon the neck, shoulders, hocks, the back and the hindquarters. Cutting horses actually pivot upon their back legs that also places a great deal of stress upon the back, hocks and the entire hindquarters. Barrel racers turn on a dime and have to possess the ability to exhibit sudden bursts of speed that predisposes them to their own unique set of stresses.

In all of these events, the use of the Thermotex™ Infrared Therapy System appliances will allow the rider, owner or trainer to have a sounder, more relaxed and comfortable animal to perform. General guidelines to follow are:

- When possible, always allow 30 – 60 minutes of warm-up with the therapy devices before an event.

Often these animals are ridden for a period of time and then prepared for their event or class. Warm the animal up before riding with a therapy session, return to the barn (stall) and then provide another therapy session before competing in the event.

• If an animal has experienced a particularly difficult day training or showing, accelerate the recovery period by providing a second therapy session later in the day.

• When these animals are stressed, provide multiple therapy sessions as needed throughout the day, each being at least 30 minutes in duration.

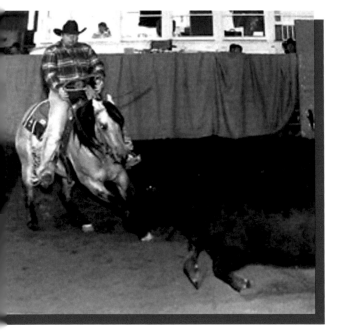

Conclusions:

There isn't a single discipline that would not benefit from therapy sessions with the Thermotex™ Infrared Therapy System appliances. Each discipline has its own unique characteristics and stresses but all can benefit from infrared heat therapy. The important fact to remember is: "These appliances provide a safe efficacious infrared heat therapy to the equine athlete. They should be used as often as practical and in as many situations as possible. They only work when they are on the horse and the only time they don't work is when they are hanging in the tack room."

Appendix A: Graphs of data averages

For detailed graphs see the efficacy study in chapter one, page 7.

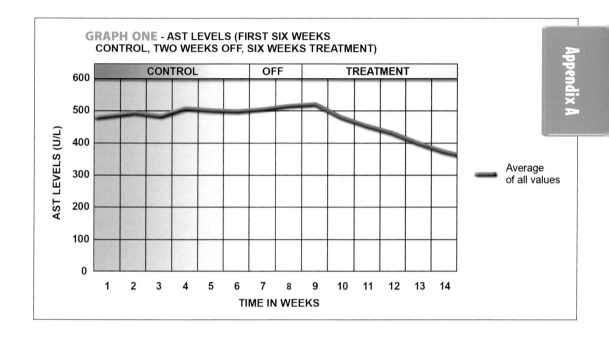

GRAPH ONE - AST LEVELS (FIRST SIX WEEKS CONTROL, TWO WEEKS OFF, SIX WEEKS TREATMENT)

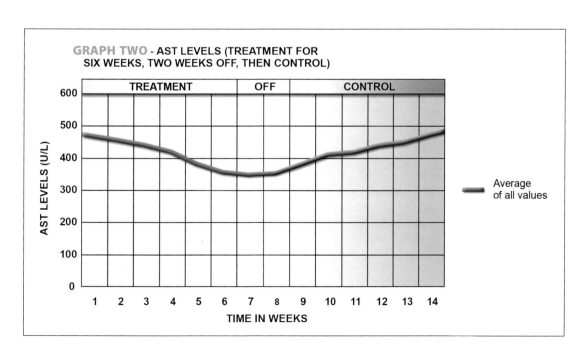

GRAPH TWO - AST LEVELS (TREATMENT FOR SIX WEEKS, TWO WEEKS OFF, THEN CONTROL)

Appendix A

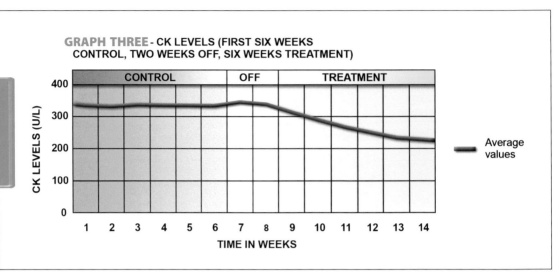

GRAPH THREE - CK LEVELS (FIRST SIX WEEKS CONTROL, TWO WEEKS OFF, SIX WEEKS TREATMENT)

CONTROL | OFF | TREATMENT

CK LEVELS (U/L)

TIME IN WEEKS

Average values

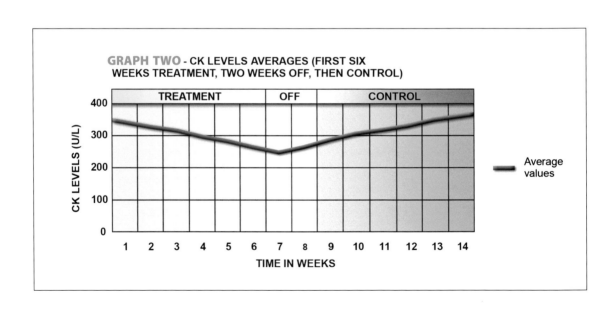

GRAPH TWO - CK LEVELS AVERAGES (FIRST SIX WEEKS TREATMENT, TWO WEEKS OFF, THEN CONTROL)

TREATMENT | OFF | CONTROL

CK LEVELS (U/L)

TIME IN WEEKS

Average values

Appendix B: Depths of temperature penetration

See research article in chapter one, page 18.

ANIMAL ONE: Temperature Measurements at Increasing Depths Over Time

DEPTH (CM)	INITIAL		5 MINUTES		10 MINUTES		15 MINUTES		20 MINUTES	
	RIGHT	LEFT	RIGHT	LEFT	RIGHT	LEFT	RIGHT	LEFT	RIGHT	LEFT
1	98.6	98.8	102.2	102	105.8	104	105.5	103.8	106.2	104.4
1.5	98.4	98.5	102.4	102.4	105.5	104.2	105.5	104	106	104
2	98.4	98.4	102.4	102.4	105.6	103.8	105.5	103.8	106.2	104
2.5	98.4	98.6	102.6	102	105.5	103	105.2	102.8	105.8	102.5
3	98.8	98.6	102.6	101.2	105.2	101	105.2	101.2	105.6	101
3.5	98.6	98.6	102.2	100.4	104.6	100.2	104.8	99.8	105.2	100.2
4	98.4	98.4	101.8	98.8	102.4	98.6	104.2	98.8	104.8	98.6
4.5	98.6	98.5	101.6	98.6	102.6	98.5	103.8	98.4	105.2	98.4
5	98.5	98.4	101.8	98.5	102.5	98.4	103.8	98.6	104.8	98.5
5.5	98.5	98.5	102	98.4	102.6	98.4	103.8	98.6	104.5	98.4
6	98.2	98.4	102.2	98.4	102.5	98.4	103.6	98.5	104.4	98.5

Appendix B

ANIMAL TWO: Temperature Measurements at Increasing Depths Over Time

DEPTH (CM)	INITIAL RIGHT	INITIAL LEFT	5 MINUTES RIGHT	5 MINUTES LEFT	10 MINUTES RIGHT	10 MINUTES LEFT	15 MINUTES RIGHT	15 MINUTES LEFT	20 MINUTES RIGHT	20 MINUTES LEFT
1	99.8	99.6	103.6	101.5	106.8	103.4	106.6	103	106.8	103.2
1.5	99.5	99.4	103.4	101.4	106.6	103.4	106.6	102.8	106.8	103
2	99.8	99.5	103.4	101.2	106.2	102.8	106.6	102.8	106.6	103.2
2.5	99.8	99.6	103.6	101.2	106.2	102	106.4	102.4	106.6	102.8
3	99.6	99.6	103.5	101.2	106.5	101.6	106.4	101.2	106.5	101
3.5	99.5	99.5	103.2	100.8	106.4	101.5	106.2	100.5	106.5	100.2
4	99.4	99.6	102.8	100.5	105.6	101.4	106.4	100.6	106.4	100.2
4.5	99.2	99.8	102.5	99.6	105.4	99.8	105.8	99.6	106.2	99.8
5	99.4	99.8	102.6	99.5	103.8	99.6	104.8	99.4	105.6	99.6
5.5	99.6	99.5	102.5	99.5	103.8	99.5	104.8	99.5	105	99.5
6	99.4	99.4	102.2	99.5	103.6	99.5	104.5	99.5	105.2	99.5

104   Appendix B

GLOSSARY

Abscess n. a pus-filled cavity resulting from inflammation and bacterial infection.

Analgesic adj. a method that alleviates pain without loss of consciousness or a type of substance that alleviates pain without loss of consciousness.

Ankylosis n. 1. the fusion of the bones of a joint, often as a result of disease or injury, or intentionally through surgery. 2. stiffness or immobility in a joint caused by bones fusing together as a result of disease or injury or arising from surgery to join one bone or part to another.

Azoturia n. an abnormal condition characterized by an excess of urea or other nitrogenous substances in the urine and by muscle damage especially to the hindquarters.

B

Bone spavin n. an inflammation of the bones in a horse's hock, resulting in swelling and lameness.

Bradykinin n. a chemical (peptide) derived from plasma protein that forms at the site of injured tissue. It plays a role in producing inflammation, dilates blood vessels and contracts smooth muscle.

Bursa n. a fluid-filled body sac that reduces friction around joints or between other parts that rub against one another.

Bursitis n. inflammation of a fluid-filled sac (bursa) of the body, particularly at the elbow, knee or shoulder joint.

C

Capped Hock n.   a soft, flabby swelling over the point of the hock caused by trauma.

Capsulitis n. an inflammation within the capsule that surrounds either an organ or part of a significant anatomical structure.

Cautery n. 1. an instrument or substance used to seal a wound or to destroy abnormal or infected tissue by burning. 2. the process or action of sealing a wound or destroying abnormal or infected tissue by burning.

Cellulitis n. infection and inflammation of the tissues beneath the skin.

Conductive adj. 1. transmitting or able to transmit energy; particularly heat or electricity. 2. used to describe a cell that allows a physiological disturbance, for example, a nerve impulse, to pass through it.

Cryosurgery n. surgery in which low temperatures are applied, for example, to destroy diseased tissue, or to seal down detached retinas.

Cunean bursa n. the bursa sac that surrounds the cunean tendon.

Cunean bursitis n. an inflammation within the cunean bursa.

D

Dehydration n. an abnormal depletion of body fluids.

Desmititis n. an inflammation within a ligament.

E

Electrocautery n. the process of destroying unwanted tissue, for example, warts and polyps, or sealing blood vessels, by means of an electrically heated needle.

Etiology n. 1. the philosophical investigation of causes and origins. 2. the branch of medicine that investigates the causes and origins of disease. 3. the set of factors that contributes to the occurrence of a disease.

G

Guttural pouch n.   these large mucous sacs are a ventral Diverticulum of the Eustachian tube and are unique to the species of the horse.

H

Hemiplegia n. total or partial inability to move, experienced on one side of the body, and caused by brain disease or injury.

Hepatic adj. 1. relating to or affecting the liver. 2. of a deep brownish-red color like that of liver.
n. any of several drugs that combat diseases of the liver.

Histamine n. an amine compound released by cells of the body's immune system in allergic reactions that causes irritation, contraction of smooth muscle, stimulation of gastric secretions, and dilation of blood vessels.

I

Inflammation n. swelling, redness, heat, and pain produced in an area of the body as a reaction to injury or infection.

Infrared n. the portion of the invisible electromagnetic spectrum consisting of radiation with wavelengths in the range 750 nm to 1mm, between light and radio waves.
adj. Using, producing, or affected by infrared radiation

Intraarticular adj. within or introduced into a joint of the body.

L

Laryngeal adj. belonging to, relating to, situated in, or affecting the larynx.

Lavage n. the washing out of a hollow body organ, for example the stomach, using a flow of water.

Lesion n. an abnormal change in the structure of a part due to injury or disease.

Ligament n. a band of fibrous tissue that connects bones or cartilages.

Lumbar adj. relating to or situated in the loins or the small of the back.

M

Modality n. something used in the treatment of a disorder.

Musculature n. 1. the way a person's or animal's muscles are arranged in a limb or organ. 2. an organism's entire muscular system.

Myoglobinuria n. an iron-containing protein resembling hemoglobin, found in muscle cells. It takes oxygen from the blood, releasing it to the muscles during strenuous exercise.

Myositis n. muscle inflammation and soreness.

N

Nebulization v to reduce a liquid to fine spray for medical use.

Neurovascular adj. of, relating to, or involving both nerves and blood vessels.

O

Osteitis n. inflammation of a bone or bony tissue, caused by infection or injury.

Osteoarthritis n. a form of arthritis characterized by gradual loss of cartilage of the joints, usually affecting people after middle age.

Osteophytes n. a small abnormal outgrowth of bone that occurs within joints or at other sites where there is degeneration of cartilage, for example, due to osteoarthritis.

P

Periostitis n. inflammation of the periosteum.

Phlebitis n. inflammation of the wall of a vein.

Prostaglandin n. an unsaturated fatty acid found in all mammals that resembles hormones in its activity, for example, controlling smooth muscle contraction, blood pressure, inflammation, and body temperature.

Protocol n. the detailed plan of a scientific experiment, medical trial, or other piece of research.

R

Renal adj. relating to or affecting the kidneys.

S

Sinus n. 1. a cavity filled with air in the bones of the face and skull, especially one opening into the nasal passages. 2. a widened channel containing blood, especially venous blood. 3. an elongated tract leading from a pus-filled region of the body to the exterior or to the cavity of a hollow organ.

Submandibular adj. relating to or located under the lower jaw.

Synovial n. a clear viscous fluid that lubricates the linings of joints and the sheaths of tendons.

Synovitis n. inflammation of the synovial membrane of a joint.

Systemic adj. 1. affecting or relating to a system as a whole. 2. affecting the whole body as distinct from having a local effect.

T

Tendonitis n. inflammation of a tendon.

Tendosynovitis n. inflammation of the tendon sheath.

Therapy n. treatment of physical, mental or behavioral problems that is meant to cure or rehabilitate somebody.

Thermograph n. 1. an instrument that continuously records temperature readings. 2. a device that shows patterns of heat radiated from a person's or an animal's body, used in diagnostic thermography.

Thoracic adj. involving or located in the chest.

Thoracolumbar adj. used to describe the thoracic and lumbar areas of the body.

V

Vasoconstriction n. narrowing of the blood vessels with consequent reduction in blood flow or increased blood pressure.

Vasodilatation n. widening of the blood vessels, especially the arteries, leading to increased blood flow or reduced blood pressure.

Viscosity n. 1. a thick and sticky consistency or quality. 2. the property of fluid or semifluid that causes it to resist flowing. 3. a measure of the resistance of a substance to motion under an applied force.